# Taught Not Caught

2

# Taught Not Caught
## strategies for sex education

**The Clarity Collective**
Helen Myles
Wendy Gale
Tricia Szirom
Deborah Davison
Sue Dyson

Illustrated by Alison Lester

British edition edited by
Hilary Dixon
Gill Mullinar

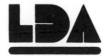

Taught Not Caught
LD405
ISBN 1 85503 046 2
© Spiral Education Resources 1983
© text The Clarity Collective 1983
© illustrations Alison Lester 1983
© illustrations on pages 113 and 114 Annabel Milne
Published under licence in the UK by LDA
All rights reserved
First Published 1985
Reprinted 1986 (twice), 1987
New Edition 1989
Reprinted 1990

Printed in England by
Ebenezer Baylis & Son Ltd
The Trinity Press, Worcester, and London

LDA, Duke Street, Wisbech, Cambs PE13 2AE

# Contents

## PREFACE TO THE SECOND BRITISH EDITION

In producing a British edition of 'Taught not Caught', we have tried above all to stay true to the spirit of the original. We have altered only those items in which the language used might have hindered comprehension, and those in which cultural and social differences rendered the activities inappropriate.

### The limitations of a Resource Book

All resources carry with them certain limitations. It is not possible, for example, to predict the exact situation in which they will be used – the degree of trust within the group, the skills of the educator, the knowledge level or maturity of the young people, or the premises in which the sessions take place. We suggest that you read the introductory section of the book and then dip into and draw from the activities in a way which is appropriate to your particular situation. No doubt 'Taught not Caught' will contain activities which you find helpful, others which you feel are less successful, and some which you cannot see yourself using at all. It is for you to exercise your judgement about the suitability of the material – the book is intended to say more about what *can* be done in sex education than what *should* be done.

### Sex Education and the Law

The Education Act (No. 2) 1986 states that governors may decide whether or not sex education shall be taught in the school. They must make and keep up to date a written statement of their policy on the content and organisation of sex education or of their decision that sex education should not form part of the curriculum.

This must be done in consultation with the Headteacher and take account of representations to them by members of the community served by the school.

This policy is normally published in the school's brochure.

There is no legal right for parents to withdraw their children from sex education. As it may be taught across many subjects or arise spontaneously in a classroom, this would be difficult. However, parents may approach the governing body with requests that their child be withdrawn from sex education on religious grounds.

Any programme of sex education will need to be developed within the policy, and teachers undertaking sex education would be wise to consult closely with senior staff.

Youth workers and others who have a responsibility for sex education outside schools will need to be familiar with current legislation and guidance, and take into account the wishes of parents where appropriate.

## Acknowledgements

We are conscious that we have been inspired, encouraged and supported by many individuals and groups in developing these strategies, and writing this book.

We would like to acknowledge the contribution made by participants in our workshop and community programmes, educators we have worked alongside, members of school committees and parent groups, and the leaders of training groups in which we have participated.

We have been particularly inspired by the work of Mary Calderone and Sol Gordon, USA, and Mary Ruth Marshall, David Merritt and Delys Sargent, Australia.

We are grateful for the encouragement and support of Anne Hanley, Lyn Horton, Wendy McCarthy, Di Mossenton, and Robin Wintle, and we owe a very special thanks to Barb Rooks for her loving support and wisdom.

For those close to us, who have lived with that often repeated phrase 'This will be the last session' – we promise *this* is!

**The Clarity Collective**

# INTRODUCTION

The Clarity Collective strongly supports education which includes the discussion and exploration of values. There is no such thing as value-free education. To state values and take a moral stand does not necessarily mean being moralistic.

We believe that moral stands such as the elimination of racism, sexism, exploitation and oppression, should be propounded in all work with young people.

The things we value and strive towards are caring, non-exploitative relationships, the opportunity to learn and grow personally, educational processes that enhance self-esteem, and the chance to share and communicate equally with the women and men in our private and working lives.

We believe we have developed some rich and exciting ways of working in sex education. This book is the way we would like to share our experiences with you.

Some years ago, we began working together as sex educators. We were employed by a family planning agency which had established an education unit to provide health and human relations education to schools, institutions and other community groups. We were all involved in planning and implementing programmes with young people, as well as providing training programmes for teachers, youth workers, nurses and other educators. We shared a common concern that, within our society, sex education is mostly left to chance learning – caught, more often than taught.

At this time, theorists were emphasising that sex education should be more than just biology, reproduction and contraceptive technology. Young people are constantly making decisions about their sexuality which incorporates how they express themselves as females and males and how they relate to others. While they do need information on topics such as sexually transmitted diseases, pregnancy, sexual preference and masturbation, this information alone does not provide them with the skills necessary to resolve day to day pressures, concerns and conflicts.

Young people want reassurance about body image, behaviour and relationships. We are convinced that the planning and presentation of sex education should encompass the opportunity for exploration of values and attitudes, and the growth of skills necessary to build relationships, communicate and make decisions.

Central to this conviction is the concept of self-esteem. A major part of human dignity is feeling good about one's self. The development of high self-esteem in young people is an essential aspect of education. If young people feel positive about themselves, they are more likely to develop non-exploitative, caring relationships, and are themselves less likely to be exploited by others.

To ensure that what we offer is relevant to young people, we have created a framework delineating the concepts, information and skills necessary to empower them so that they may be more in control of decisions that affect their lives.

Self-esteem is the core of our framework, so all our strategies are designed to be esteem building.

This book is the integration of our philosophy and practical experience. It is influenced by our feminism and our belief that the development of sexuality should be a positive part of personal growth.

# Part A
# The framework

# The framework

When you are working with young people in sex education you need a theoretical and philosophical framework.

It is established that young women have lower levels of self-esteem during adolescence than young men, and this places them at a disadvantage. The sexist assumptions of much sex education reinforce and maintain this disadvantage. That young women are more passive in sexual relationships than young men, that women are responsible for contraception, that women are physically weaker, or that women will be the homemakers and men the breadwinners are examples of sexist assumptions expressed in some sex education teaching and resources.

A purely heterosexist approach to sex education ignores the fact that by no means all sexual orientations are towards the opposite sex. It is important to recognise that perhaps one person in ten may be homosexual in any group. An increase in understanding of homosexuality among the rest of the group may also be important.

The following framework takes into account these and other factors regarding the nature and expression of sexuality.

Sexuality is an integral part of life and it influences personality. It may be denied, repressed or used effectively but it is part of our selves. Sexuality is a process commencing at birth and ending only with death. For every person there are significant events which highlight sexuality. These include puberty, menopause, choosing a partner or partners and childbirth. Sexuality is culturally defined and thus influenced by family, peers, religion, economics, school, media, law and science. The way people feel about themselves determines the way they express their sexuality. The relationships in which people express their sexuality are many and varied. In society we will encounter, in addition to heterosexuality, preferences which include celibacy, bisexuality and homosexuality. For some people, these preferences may change during their lives.

**Building the framework**

*figure 1*

Birth
Puberty
Menopause
Death

Sexuality is a life-long process. There are specific events which are significant to our sexuality. This is demonstrated on the framework by drawing a lifeline and marking in these significant events.

This framework focuses on the period beginning with puberty and extending into young adulthood.

5

# The framework

figure 2

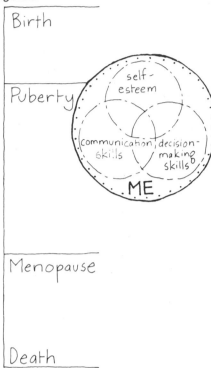

Each young person, represented as ME, arrives at puberty bringing the sum of their life's experience to that point. This includes self-esteem, communication and decision-making skills. These are represented on the framework by three overlapping circles demonstrating their inter-related nature. *Self-esteem* is a concept about self which incorporates how a person feels about her or his body and the pleasure that can be derived from it. At puberty many young people, particularly young women, experience a drop in their feelings of self-worth, so when working with them be aware of the need to constantly build their self-esteem. Self-esteem influences everything people do; their communication and decision-making skills hinge upon it.

Many young people have not had the opportunity to develop *communication skills* necessary to express their thoughts, fears, hopes and ideas or to question. Incorporate ways of developing verbal, non-verbal and inter-personal skills throughout your work.

*The ability to make decisions* is critical. During our lives there are many decisions to be made related to sexuality. For many people these turn out to be non-decisions because they don't know the options, and don't have the opportunity to discuss actions and their consequences. Decisions are often made under emotional pressure, so it is important to provide opportunities to learn the skill of decision making without these pressures.

figure 3

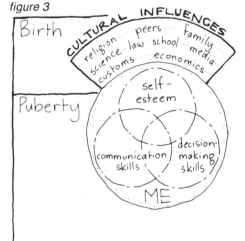

All of us exist within certain parameters which define the ways in which we can grow. These parameters include *customs, the family, economics, peers, the law, the media, science, religion and school.* Young people are particularly susceptible to the influence of these institutions. They affect the way young people feel about themselves, their decision-making processes, the way they communicate, the information they receive and the formation of their concepts and values.

It is important to acknowledge the influence of these parameters. This can be done through activities which explore the influence of the media, family and peers, or by constantly referring to the ways in which we develop our values and attitudes.

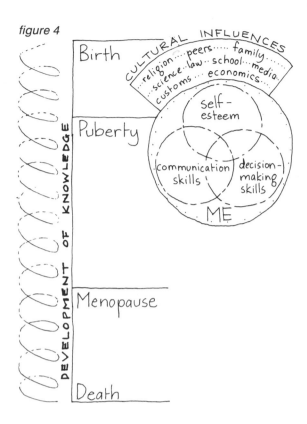

figure 4

Young people bring with them to puberty a *body of knowledge.* This is indicated on the framework as a spiral because learning occurs throughout life and is comprised of facts and life experience. The acquisition and use of knowledge is a factor which determines whether sexuality is a constructive or destructive force. Young people need to have adequate knowledge in time to influence sexual decision making. When planning, ascertain the level of knowledge in the group and make sure that the activities you use reflect the participants' needs.

From puberty onwards there are certain decisions to be made relating to sexuality. These decisions may not be permanent. In light of changing circumstances, different environments, new knowledge and experience, decisions can be changed and revoked and new ones made. Decisions are not made in isolation — one stems from another, and each one has a ripple effect on other aspects of life. Decisions include choosing a partner or partners, marriage, living together, casual relationships, monogamy, quality of relationships, and degrees of commitment.

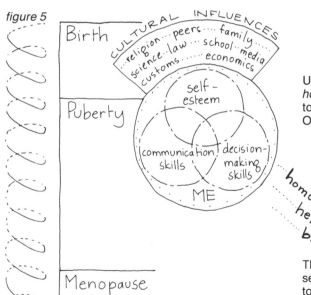

figure 5

Underlying all sexual decision making are feelings of either *homosexuality or heterosexuality.* Young people will have to make decisions about whether or not to act on these. Once made, the decisions are not irrevocable.

The choice of sexual preference, to be homosexual, heterosexual or bisexual is one which can be reassessed from time to time. For some, however, it will be a permanent decision.

## The framework

figure 6

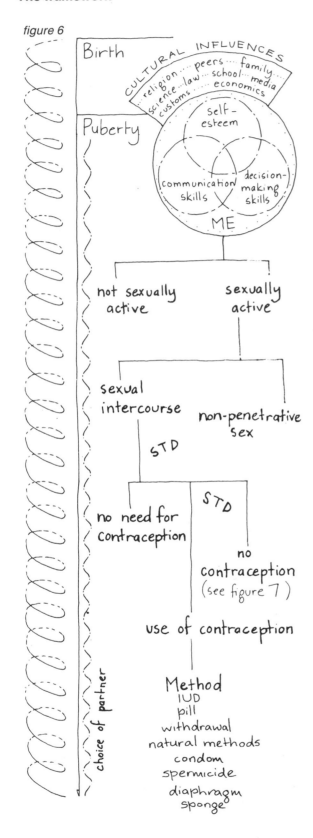

The first specific decision to be made is whether to be *sexually active or not.* At certain points in their lives some people make a decision to be *celibate.* That is, they consciously decide not to be sexually active. Sexual activity includes kissing, masturbation, petting, and the like.

The next decision will be whether or not to have *sexual intercourse.* Many do not recognise that young people are sexually active. By the time they are 19, a large number of them will be having sexual intercourse. They are under a lot of pressure from their peers and the media to become sexually active, so it is important to be aware of these factors and address these issues.

The risk of contracting a *sexually transmitted disease* (STD) can come at any time on the lifeline after the decision to become sexually active. It is important to raise the issue of responsibility to self and others, obtaining treatment and informing sexual contacts.

If the decision has been to have heterosexual intercourse, the next step is to decide if *contraception* will be used or not. In order to make the decision to use contraception, young people have to admit to themselves that they are having sexual intercourse. They will need to know where to go to obtain contraception. It is desirable for them to be able to talk to their partner or partners, and parents for support and advice.

If contraception is decided upon, the next decision is which *method* to use. Many young people have a limited knowledge of effective methods. They can also feel embarrassed and inhibited when seeking contraception. These barriers need to be overcome for young people to be effective users of contraception.

8

*figure 7*

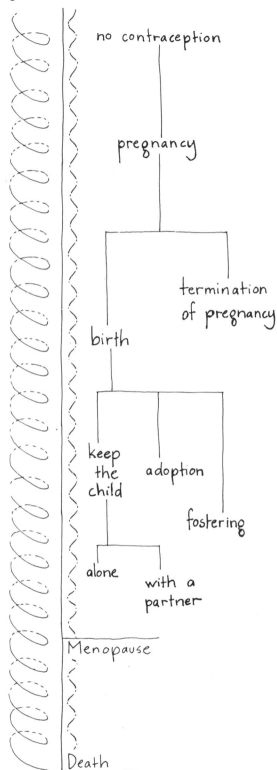

If the decision is not to use contraception there will be a high risk of *pregnancy.* Some young people do not use contraception because they believe they will not get pregnant.

Should pregnancy occur, the next decision is to either *terminate the pregnancy* or *maintain it.* A large number of young women have their pregnancies terminated. This is not an easy decision. Unwanted pregnancies highlight the necessity for sound contraceptive education.

Maintaining the pregnancy requires a choice from three options — *adoption, fostering* or *keeping the child.*

If the decision is to keep the child it will be necessary to make a further decision to remain *alone* or be with a *partner.* This is particularly relevant at this time, but the decision to *choose a partner* is one which can be made at various points on the lifeline. This is shown by a wavy line parallel to the lifeline from puberty on.

**This framework is dynamic. It will continually evolve and develop as you work with it. This whole book is based on this framework and courses can be built around it.**

## The framework

figure 8

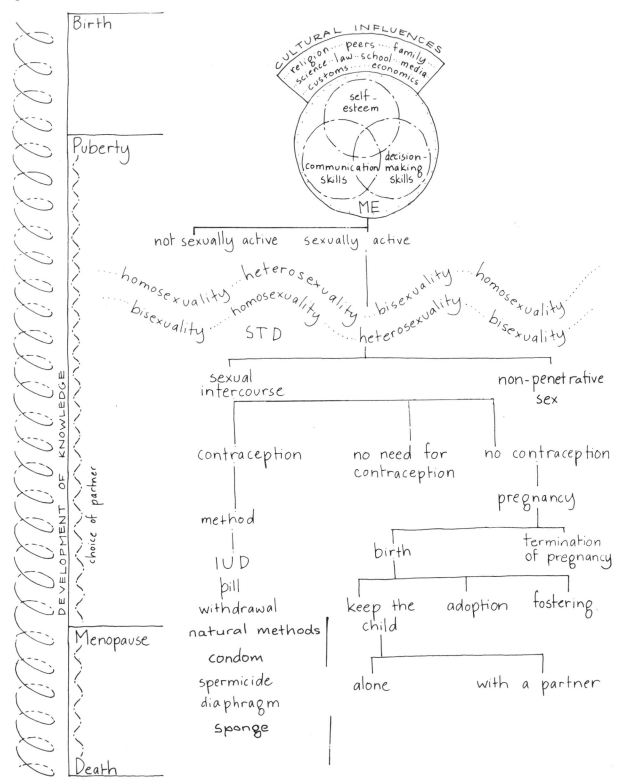

# PART B
# Preparation

# Section 1
# You as the educator

**The most important tool in sex education is the educator. It is essential to spend a lot of time preparing yourself before you start working in this area. There are several questions you need to consider.**

### 1 Why am I involved in sex education?
You may be involved in sex education for a variety of reasons: you may be specifically employed to teach the subject, it might have been delegated to you, perhaps you believe that young people have a right to information. Whatever your reason for being involved, examine your personal motives — what you hope to achieve from your involvement for yourself and others.

### 2 Where do I stand?
Sex education is not, and cannot be, value free, but you can be aware of your values and lessen the chance of imposing your biases on the people with whom you work. It is essential to consider your own stand on certain issues before undertaking work in this area, because this can influence the way you present material and ideas.

### 3 What are my supports?
Working in a team provides an ideal support system. However, you may find yourself in the isolated position of being the only one providing sex education where you work, or you may feel that there is no support for what you are doing. It is important to have people around you to back you up, share ideas, motivate and challenge you. Approach sympathetic and like-minded people from your staff, parents' groups, management bodies and the general community to establish a support group. Parents and community members are an under-utilised resource. Other sources of support are health centres, school nurses, family planning clinics, local health education officers, local NCT groups, nursing mothers, rape crisis centres and women's health groups. You could then draw on this support group to help plan, present and evaluate your work. By involving a wide range of people you will not be alone in teaching what may be a controversial area.

It is useful to attend as many workshops and courses as possible. As well as exposing yourself to new ideas, techniques and strategies, you will be able to develop a broader network of support. One advantage of working in a team is that members can attend a range of workshops, then pool and share their learning.

### 4  Why include some topics and not others?
Reasons for including some topics and not others may be lack of time, insufficient knowledge and resources, group interests or agency policy. However, you may find yourself saying that 'the group isn't ready yet', when in fact it may be your own unrecognised feelings of inadequacy and discomfort. You need to acknowledge your feelings, accept them, and work towards feeling more comfortable with the topic.

Some ways of doing this are to work in pairs or teams; to involve other people to cover areas where you lack knowledge or feel uncomfortable, by inviting speakers from appropriate agencies; to increase your information base through reading, working together, and attending courses; and to work through areas of discomfort or embarrassment by yourself or with others.

### 5  What language will be used?
Language you will encounter may range from technical jargon, to slang, to baby talk. There is a great deal of power in language, and most young people are not familiar with technical terminology. This puts them at a disadvantage. It may be appropriate to start by clarifying colloquial words. See *There's another name for it* (page 111) and decide with the group through discussion what language is appropriate and acceptable for the session or course.

In any group of young people there may be some who are sexually active while others are not. Never assume knowledge, experience or sexual preference. Phrases like 'when you start having intercourse . . .' assume that no one is yet sexually active. A more appropriate statement might be: 'Some people in this group may need this information now, and most of you will need it at some time in your life . . .'

Be aware that language maintains sexism: always referring to doctors as 'he' implies that all doctors are male. Language also maintains heterosexism: that is, it validates the assumption that sexual relationships are always between members of the opposite sex. Permanent relationships are almost always discussed in terms of wife and husband.

Use language with care and remove sexist and heterosexist terms to include a wider range of people in discussions. The recognition that sexist and heterosexist language excludes some people is an important part of sex education.

### 6  What knowledge is needed?
Many areas of education require the educator to be an expert. This is not so in this field. Reproduction information has often been presented as the sole component of sex education. Reproduction is an important component, but other factors such as values and concepts are of equal importance. Sexuality incorporates how people express themselves as females and males, including how they relate to others, so an understanding of the concepts involved in communicating and relationships is essential. However, a sound knowledge of facts about the body, contraception, sexually transmitted diseases, pregnancy and birth is important and will provide you with confidence to answer questions.

At the beginning of each new subject area in this book there is a Fact Sheet. For an example see page 67. The Fact Sheets include information to help with preparation, and materials for use in your work. By considering the factors presented, knowing and understanding the words and reading the references to gain a breadth of knowledge and opinion, you will be adequately prepared.

It is also important to be familiar with the questions commonly asked by young people.

What happens during an abortion?

How do you know when you've got an STD?

How do you get AIDS?

Can you explain how to use tampons?

When do you take the pill, before or after?

What is circumcision and why do it?

Do men or boys have anything like periods?

What is a wet dream?

Do all girls bleed when the hymen is broken? If so, does it hurt?

What is an orgasm?

What is carnal knowledge?

What is a D and C?

There are some other commonly asked questions that may require more than facts for answers.

What does randy mean?

What does it mean when a girl is called frigid?

Should you be a virgin before marriage?

How can I tell if I'm really in love?

Is sexual intercourse painful?

What do lesbians do when they have sex?

How do you know if you are a homosexual?

Only gays get AIDS don't they?

My girlfriend is pregnant, what shall we do?

Is it normal to masturbate?

Can you get pregnant from heavy petting?

Can you get contraception without your parents knowing?

How do you say no?

Why should women have to worry about rape, sexual pressures and getting pregnant when men have all the fun?

15

If you are unable to answer a question, acknowledge this and work with the group to gain this knowledge.

Attending relevant courses will be of enormous value and the knowledge gained will enhance the use of the activities in this book.

Keep in touch with relevant current affairs and be familiar with television programmes watched by your group. These are important sources of issues which are sure to be raised by enquiring young people.

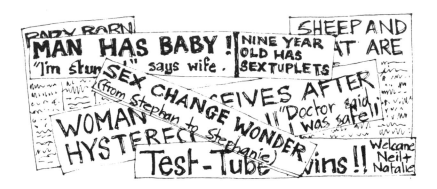

### 7  How will I deal with unexpected situations?

Unexpected situations will always arise. At some stage you will have to deal with a situation such as the film not arriving, the projector breaking down or the guest speaker arriving late. Sometimes an activity may not work or is completed in a much shorter time than expected. Always have an alternative activity planned. You should also consider your reaction to the stress of such an event.

Another difficult situation may be that participants ask for personal opinions or intimate details of your own life. In order to respond appropriately it may help to consider the questioner's possible motives. They may want to know more about you; want fuel for confrontation with parents; want to reinforce their own opinions; be testing you; or they may want to avoid their own decision-making. Responses will vary according to the membership, age and size of the group, the length of time you are together, the topic, and what you want to achieve. Consider the context in which you are working and how supportive this is of personal sharing. You cannot expect others in the group to give of themselves if you don't.

## 8 What makes a good working environment?

A warm, friendly environment enhances sex education. One aspect of the environment is the room to be used for the session. The way the room is physically structured can either limit or enhance group interaction. Whenever possible check on the room prior to planning the session. Decide what it is you want to achieve and set up the room accordingly.

If it is a formal lecture, panel or film, ensure that everyone can see and hear properly.

If you want to have an informal discussion don't attempt it with the participants sitting in rows. Stack the tables and arrange the chairs in a circle. Many centres have a room set aside for discussion groups and have furnished these with carpet and comfortable chairs.

If you can't modify the room, change your position for presentation. For example, work from the back of the room, or sit on a desk. These establish new environments for the session.

If you have no choice about the facilities available, adapt or use activities that are appropriate to your environment — intimate group discussion is difficult in a science laboratory.

## 9 How do I work with the group?

Developing trust

The role of the educator is to establish a climate of trust and acceptance within the group. This means working first on trust-building activities and leaving factual and more involved subjects until later sessions. With a friendly and accepting group it is possible to explore personal issues and have greater participation from all.

When a good climate exists, members will feel comfortable to participate in their own way. Whenever possible, and appropriate, allow them to choose their own small groupings so that they will not be allocated to groups in which they feel uncomfortable or self-conscious. It is possible for you to check the feelings of the group by answering a few questions.

Is there trust and honesty between all members, including the educator?

Is there a feeling of care and concern within the group?

Do all members feel a sense of belonging?

Is there co-operation?

Does everyone have the opportunity to contribute and to try new things?

Some basic factors to consider for developing a climate of trust are: establishing contracts, confidentiality, consistency and the use of non-threatening and non-competitive strategies and techniques which build, rather than diminish self-esteem.

At the commencement of a course, the educator needs to establish modes of mutually acceptable behaviour with the group. This is sometimes called setting contracts. The areas in which contracts can be set are: confidentiality, respect for others, not ridiculing each other, observing the right to pass, the validity of all comments, the right to negotiate subject matter and assessment.

Confidentiality was summed up by one young woman who said, 'If you say it here, hear it here, or do it here, leave it here.'

Consistency is the key to developing trust. Keep your word. If you have established a contract, stick to it.

### How people behave in groups

In all groups, formal and informal rules about acceptable behaviour apply. These are group norms. It is important for you to recognise the group norms that affect work in this area. The norm that does not allow group members to talk about their personal feelings will hinder meaningful discussion. This attitude can be diffused in several ways: by changing the physical environment; by establishing a contract that during the time the group is together, new rules apply; or by establishing more formal and explicit rules.

For formal rules to be effective, members need to participate equally and fully in their formulation, acknowledge that new rules exist and feel committed to carrying them out.

Finally, in preparing yourself, consider the following guidelines:

Respect the rights of the individual group members.

Encourage participants to respond honestly.

Provide an atmosphere that encourages diversity of opinion.

Attempt to be accepting and non-judgemental.

Develop active listening skills.

Work at the three levels of facts, concepts and attitudes so that broader social issues are addressed.

Develop a sense of humour.

# Section 2
# Techniques

**Techniques are methods of working with a group. All the techniques you will need to effectively conduct the activities are included in this section.**

### Group Discussion

Group discussion does not require elaborate equipment and resources. It is a valuable technique to use in sex education. Of all the skills and resources available, the ability to clarify, question, explain, draw out and sum up is the most important. Effective use of these skills provides the opportunities for groups and individuals to discuss the issues for themselves.

Group size affects participation. If there are more than fifteen in a group, involvement may be reduced. Divide large groups into smaller groups of 3 or 4 for more effective discussions. The educator should move from group to group providing assistance whenever necessary. Allow time for small groups to share a summary of their discussion with the large group.

Set up the room so that all members can see and hear properly. They should be comfortable and facing each other. It can be intimidating to be confronted with a large circle of chairs in an otherwise empty room. It is more effective to ask the group to rearrange the room themselves.

Triggers such as videos or films, guest speakers, television programmes and newspaper articles can be used to initiate discussion.

The discussion will work if you have set yourself clear objectives. You can lead a group through a complete topic in a logical sequence by presenting new points to the group when necessary.

Be conscious of individuals who may dominate the discussion; provide opportunities for quiet members to speak and attempt to draw them out. If you have a contract ensuring the right to pass, it is important to allow people to retain that right. Ask clarifying questions, and sum up discussion at regular intervals as well as at the conclusion.

**Techniques**

Silence is important. It will be helpful to explain this to the group. If the discussion leader is comfortable with silence, valuable reflection time can occur.

**Structured Group Discussion**

Sometimes it is useful to use structured methods to stimulate discussion when the topic is controversial or to encourage the expression of a wide range of views. Three suggested methods are Fishbowl, Hot Seat, and Debates.

**Fishbowl** Introduce the topic. Set up two circles of seating — an outer circle for observers, and an inner one for the fishbowl. This technique can be used with a group of any size, but the fishbowl should consist of 7 to 10 people.

Two groups volunteer to become particpants in the fishbowl. One group is to speak in favour of the topic and the other against. It is optional to give the group time to prepare. Set a time limit of 5 to 10 minutes for each group to present its case, and an overall time limit of 30 minutes for the activity.

One group goes into the fishbowl together to present its position. The other group remain observers until it is their turn. Members of each group present their points without debate or argument.

After both teams have presented their positions, the fishbowl is thrown open. This means that the observers can join the fishbowl by tapping one of the fishbowl members on the shoulder and taking that place. At this time individuals can put their points of view, discuss and argue the issues. If discussion seems to be lagging, close the fishbowl early.

**The Hot Seat** This is a variation of a fishbowl. A spare chair is placed in the fishbowl circle. If anyone sits in that chair they have the right to make one statement without challenge. The person can only make one statement from the chair and then must move back into the large circle or the fishbowl.

**Debates** When using debates it is not always necessary to use strict rules; just use the concept of debating in teams.
See *A progressive debate* (page 161).

## Brainstorming

Brainstorming is a creative way of generating the greatest number of ideas in the shortest possible time. It allows for maximum group participation. It can be used to generate common definitions and terminology and to plan courses and activities. It can also be used in groups as an ice-breaker or where individuals find it hard to contribute.

For brainstorming to be successful it is imperative to abide by three simple rules.

1 Accept every idea uncritically and write it down.

2 Aim for quantity not quality.

3 No discussion.

The procedure is very simple. Decide on a topic or issue. State the topic clearly to the group. Appoint one or two participants to list the ideas as they are called out. The lists must be clearly visible to all.

State the rules clearly and enforce them as brainstorming proceeds. Restate the topic. Set and enforce a time limit of about 10 minutes. At the end of the set time, go through the list and code the responses. For example, they could cross out all the impossible or unrealistic suggestions, put a star against the ones they would use, tick the ones they want to know more about, underline those not understood by all the group. Allow time for general discussion.

The large group may form smaller groups to use this technique. Reform the large group to share responses at the end.

## Values clarification

All people, especially young people, are constantly bombarded with conflicting messages about what to do, think and feel. They are often confused by this, and uncertain about which message is right. The media, school, parents, friends and religion may present different versions about what is 'right'. Ultimately young people must be able to decide this for themselves.

To aid this process, a technique called values clarification has been developed. This approach is not about the content of values, but about creating a process whereby young people can begin to learn the skill of deciding what they value and making choices and decisions. Once this skill has been learned it can be applied throughout life. Some examples of values which young people may clarify in sex education are trust, love, honesty, chastity, independence, integrity, belonging and respect.

However, when choosing the techniques to use, be aware that values clarification is not always the most appropriate. If you want to convince or persuade, then don't use values clarification. For example, do not use it if you are trying to convince a group that rape is wrong.

The values clarification process is based on the work of Louis Raths, and has been developed by a number of others, principally Sidney Simon. According to him, the valuing process consists of seven sub-processes.

Choosing one's beliefs and behaviours:

1  Choosing from alternatives.

2  Choosing after considering the consequences.

3  Choosing freely.

Prizing one's beliefs and behaviours:

4  Prizing and cherishing.

5  Publicly affirming, when appropriate.

Acting on one's beliefs:

6  Acting.

7  Acting with a pattern consistently and with repetition.[1]

This approach does not offer a set of values that are 'right', but enables people to gain insight into those beliefs that influence their behaviour, choices and decisions.

Sometimes when using values clarification it is necessary to play the role of devil's advocate. A group may be so homogenous that they fail to consider all the aspects available to them during a values clarification activity. In this situation the educator can openly state 'I think I could put a case for . . .' and thus broaden the options open to the participants.

The way the values clarification technique is presented for use in this book is as activities that raise issues, enabling people to sort out their own personal values at their own pace. Look under Values Clarification in the activity index for examples.

Values clarification helps people develop the skills they need to sort out the chaos and complexity of life, and to choose the things they value. This is particularly significant in learning about and dealing with one's sexuality.

Exploring one's attitudes is difficult. It needs patience and support.

[1] Simon, Sidney et al, *Values Clarification A Handbook of Practical Strategies for Teachers and Students*, Hart Publishing Co, NY, 1978.

**Problem-solving and decision-making**

Life is full of problems and decisions, and many people do not have the appropriate skills to manage them. These skills are able to be learnt. Solving problems and making decisions may be an individual or a group process, but it is important to see it as a process.

When looking at a problem, it is necessary to identify the core problem and whose it is. Examine all sides of the question. Establish and obtain the relevant facts. Consider the range of possible alternatives and examine the implications of each alternative. Make a decision, based on the steps identified and the information collected. Adherence to a group decision will be most effective if there is concensus among group members.

A useful way to develop problem-solving and decision-making skills is to present a dilemma situation. This simulates a process that can be used in real-life situations. An example of a dilemma situation is *Jenny's dilemma* (page 85).

**Role-play**

Role-play is not new. We do it all our lives, starting as children playing mothers and fathers. Role-play is also an educational technique which allows the participants to play themselves in different or unknown situations, such as school students preparing for job interviews; to play the part of another person in a known situation, such as reversing roles so that students become teachers or children become parents; and to play other people in unknown situations, such as fantasy games or historical enactments.

By using role-play as an educational technique, emotions, reactions, thoughts, behaviours, attitudes and values can be explored. At the end of the role-play, participants can reflect on the experience, and gain greater understanding of the given situations.

Role-play has limitations. It cannot solve all problems, and it depends heavily on the participants' abilities to be creative.

On the other hand, it has potential. It can be used as a base for discussion; it can increase communication skills and self-esteem; it demonstrates other situations and ways of dealing with them; and it allows participants to see how others feel in a given situation. The shared experience of a role-play can bring the group close together.

When using role-play, have clear and well defined objectives. Involve everyone, as participants with a role, or as observers.

Allow about one-fifth of the total session time for preparing the group. This is essential to create the mood and encourage participants to feel relaxed. Use movement activities which stimulate imagination and creativity. An example of a warm-up is *Building a machine* (page 53).

Ask participants to volunteer for the various roles, but never force people into roles they do not want to play. Use costumes, hats, name tags and other props to identify participants in their roles if this is felt to be helpful.

Encourage participants to identify with the role they are playing. If they are playing an unknown character, ask them to respond in the way they think that person would. If they are playing themselves in an unknown situation, ask them to respond as honestly as possible to that situation.

You should not assume that role-play will run by itself. You need to stage manage and direct it. Keep encouraging the players to remain in the role and fully explore the situation.

Prepare observers by handing out observation sheets with questions such as:

What sort of people were they?    What feelings were expressed?

What happened?                            How did the others react?

Why did it happen?

Deroling is as important as role preparation. At the end of the role-play, before any discussion, give all the players an opportunity to express their feelings about the characters and situations they portrayed. Then all the role players shed their characters by removing any identifying symbols. It may also be necessary to have everyone change seats or identify themselves by their real name and say something about themselves. Do not underestimate the need for this. Deroling is then complete and players should no longer be referred to in character either by reference or name.

Debriefing is the period when valuable reflection and evaluation occurs. Ensure there is sufficient time for this. As themselves, the players discuss what they learned from the experience. Ask observers to contribute to the analysis of the role-play and encourage general discussion about the relevance of the situation to their lives.

### Quizzes

A quiz can be verbal or written. When used in sex education, a quiz can be an enjoyable way of imparting new information, reinforcing knowledge and correcting misinformation. It may help educators and students decide the content of a course. It can also be used as a discussion starter.

An essential component for the educator using a quiz is a thorough knowledge of the facts being tested. In answering quiz questions there are often opportunities for the educator to impart new information to a receptive group, so a high level of knowledge is a necessary prerequisite.

The answer sheets provided with the quizzes in this book, give brief answers with no detail. It is essential to expand these with information gained from the references.

For the quiz to be most beneficial as an educational tool, all aspects of testing should be removed and the element of fun retained.

### Videos or films

Most young people enjoy and respond to videos. There is a wide range of relevant and informative videos available which can enhance sex education. If you use videos, follow them with relevant activities which will clarify and offer additional information, explore values and attitudes, and provide opportunities for young people to share their opinions and feelings.

Some suggested follow-up activities:

After viewing the video re-arrange the room to allow face to face participation in group discussion (page 19).

At the end of the video, and before any discussion, ask individuals to write their reactions and feelings about it. Then ask participants to form small groups to share and compare their reactions. Allow time for total group sharing if appropriate.

Role-play (page 23) can be used to complement or expand a video. Have the group act out a range of other possible endings for it.

Prepare a questionnaire that reviews the content of the video.

Use I feel . . . (page 134) to gain a group reaction.

Always preview the video. Titles, and even synopses, can be misleading; fact and content can be incorrect and out of date. Know why you are using it and what you hope the group will gain. Be aware that the video may be appropriate for several topic areas, not just the stated title. Be in control. Interrupt the screening if it is appropriate. Even if you have seen the video several times, it is important to stay in the room to gauge the reaction of that particular group. It may be advantageous to show it more than once in a course to clarify items that may have been missed or not understood.

### Visiting speakers

To supplement a sex education course it can be useful to involve visiting speakers. Be aware that there are some limitations. The speaker may present a one-sided view on the subject; you will not be familiar with their skill in presentation and you are dependent on them to present their information. Therefore, if necessary, invite a variety of speakers to cover different aspects of a topic, contact the speaker to familiarise yourself with the style and content to be used, and always have an alternative activity planned in the event that the speaker does not arrive.

There are many benefits to be gained from having a visiting speaker. Contact with a person who has broader experience and specialised knowledge gives the participants an opportunity to gain insight into, and understanding of this experience. Visiting speakers can be part of the educator's support system and if you feel unfamiliar with a subject, a guest speaker can provide you with a role model for future presentations, and at the same time, the participants get the information which you are unable to provide.

The educator needs to be present during the guest speaker's session, so that in subsequent sessions you can supplement knowledge, clarify areas of uncertainty, discuss reactions to the material presented and develop the topic further.

Brief the speaker prior to the visit by placing the session in context. Clarify mutual expectations, including the specific role that you will play during the session. It is also necessary to establish the resources needed and have them ready for the session.

Group members should be involved in the planning and organising of the session for guest speakers. For an example of how to involve the participants see *Breast feeding* (page 163).

# Section 3
# Planning and evaluation

### Planning

The planning process is the same whether it is for a single activity, a session or a course. An effective plan will be realistic, logical and sequential, as well as being consistent with the needs and interests of the participants and appropriate to the educational context. Showing videos or using activities merely because they may be enjoyable could indicate inadequate planning or a lack of clear objectives.

The first task when planning is to identify objectives. These can be stated in terms of behaviour, facts, concepts and values. The focus of the objectives should be the participants and what they will achieve. The objectives must be realistic. Participants will have a clearer idea of why they are participating and the outcome of that participation if you state and discuss the objectives at the beginning of each course, session or activity.

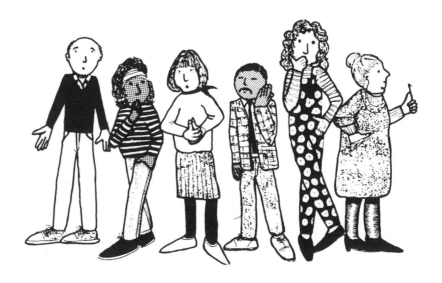

# Course Planner

| Why objectives | What? session title | How? activity | When? date & time | Where? location | Who? team members resource people | How? evaluation |
|---|---|---|---|---|---|---|
| | | | | | | |

Permission to copy this page for participant use

28

# Planning and evaluation

Consult with participants and involve them from the beginning when planning. Do not automatically accept the word of adults about what young people want to know. Each group is different and their experience is valid. Use *Brainstorming* (page 21) or *Setting objectives and priorities* (page 33) to identify the learning needs of the group.

A major problem in planning is the time factor. Consider the time available realistically, and set priorities so that the most important objectives can be achieved.

Discuss the following questions with your support group or team: why? what? how? when? where? and who? If you are planning a course the answers to these questions will provide the components and will enable you to fill out the Course Planner (page 28). Remember that even after a plan has been drawn up, it can still be altered to suit the changing needs of the group.

If you are planning a whole course and you have completed the Course Planner you will need to plan the details of each session. This will ensure that the content is covered in the time allowed. For an example of a Session Planner see below.

| Session Planner | | | |
|---|---|---|---|
| OBJECTIVE | At the end of this session participants will be able to demonstrate knowledge about body changes at puberty and the reasons these occur. | | |
| TIME | ACTIVITY | EQUIPMENT | PERSON RESPONSIBLE |
| 10.00 | *Changes* (page 131) | large sheets of paper, felt-tip pens | S.D. |
| 10.45 | theory input on changes to the body at puberty | overhead projector, charts | W.G. |
| 11.05 | *Puberty quiz* (page 137) | copies of quiz (page 138) answers | W.G. |
| 11.40 | Evaluation *Field of words* (page 37) | writing materials, copy of *Field of words* (38) | S.D. |
| 11.50 | session finish | | |
| EVALUATION METHOD | Assessment through the quiz will measure the participants' knowledge of the subject. The field of words will indicate the participants' reactions to the session. | | |

### Choosing and using an activity

Given that an activity is specifically designed to highlight the content and to assist in achieving your aims, ask yourself why you are including a particular activity. Recognise that activities are a means to an end, not an end in themselves, and fit them into the context of the session. Understand the activity fully before you use it. Learn the rules, familiarise yourself with any variations and be aware of the pitfalls which may occur during it. If you are working with someone else, become familiar with the activity together beforehand. Make sure you both know exactly which sections each is handling. Practise giving the instructions out aloud. Detailed instructions can be presented from a sheet, but if you choose to do this don't hide the fact — do it openly. Be flexible and change the activity if necessary. Be careful not to change it without direction and an understanding of how to finish appropriately. Stay involved, even if you've done the activity dozens of times before.

At the completion of an activity invite participants to discuss their feelings about participating in it, how they feel after some reflection and what they have learnt. This debriefing period is necessary to assess the effectiveness of the activity from both your own and the participants' point of view. This is one way of establishing if the activity has achieved its objectives, and if not, why not.

The activities in this book are in a sequence which could be followed when planning, but this is not essential. You can use similar activities to achieve different aims, in different subject areas and as you become more experienced you can make up your own activities.

### Evaluation

Evaluation is the means by which you establish not only how effective you have been as an educator, but also the direction the group is taking and whether your choice of teaching method is appropriate. It enables the participants to assess their learning for themselves and it is also a method of establishing accountability for a course. Evaluation is a planning tool from which you set new objectives.

Assessment should not be confused with evaluation. Assessment is only part of the evaluation process. The quizzes and questionnaires included in this book will help you assess the participants' level of information. They can also provide you with feedback about your teaching effectiveness, but they cannot indicate to what extent individuals have participated, what the major concerns were, or what attitudes and behaviours have been affected. It is possible to evaluate yourself and your work by directly asking the participants or others by asking the questions in *Evaluation voting* (page 35), by distributing the *Review sheets* (pages 40 and 41), or by personal observation.

The first eight activities in this book are concerned with planning and evaluation.

# Part C
# Activities

# Planning and evaluation

**References:**
Allen, I., *Education in Sex and Personal Relationship*, Policy Studies Institute, 1987
Button, L., *Developmental Group Work with Adolescents*, Hodder and Stoughton, 1974
Dallas, D. M., *Sex Education in School and Society*, NFER 1972
David, K. and Williams, T. (eds.), *Health Education in Schools*, Harper and Row, 1987
Farrell, C., *My Mother Said*, Routledge & Kegan Paul, 1978
H.M. Inspectorate, *Health Education from 5-16*, HMSO, 1986
Lee, C., *The Ostrich Position: Sex, Schooling and Mystification*, Unwin, 1986
Massey, D., *School Sex Education: Why What and How*, FPA Education Unit, 1988
National Council of Women, *Sex education — Whose Responsibility?*, National Council for Women, 1984
Nottinghamshire County Council, *Report by Working Party on Sex Education in Schools*, Nottinghamshire Advisory & Inspection Service, 1979
Rogers, R. S. (ed.), *Sex Education, Rationale and reaction*, Cambridge University Press, 1974
Taylor, B., *Experimental Learning: a Framework for Group Skills*, Oasis Publications, 2 St. Mary's, Bootham, York, 1983
Went, D. J., *Sex Education: Some Guidelines for Teachers*, Bell & Hyman, 1985

**Videos/Films**
Developmental Work with Tutorial Groups
It's Sex Next Week
Let's Talk About It

**Additional Resources**
Childhood
Family Lifestyles
Health Action Pack
Health Matters

**Activities**
1  Setting objectives and priorities
2  Sentence stems
3  Evaluation voting
4  Evaluation ranking
5  Evaluation — field of words
6  Review sheets
   Form A   Review sheet for the end of a session
   Form B   Review sheet for the end of a unit
7  Telemessages
8  Evaluation collage

# 1 Setting objectives and priorities

**Objectives**          To introduce the idea of self-directed learning.
To gain information from the group for course planning.
To make the content of the course relevant to as many group members as possible.

**Prerequisites**       Literacy skills.

**Age group**           13-16, 16 +
This activity could be adapted for 9-13 year olds.

**Group size**          Ideally a maximum of 25.

**Time needed**         30-45 minutes.

**What you need**       Personal writing materials, paper, felt-tip pens.

**How you do it**

a  Ask each person to write down privately what she or he would like to learn, know more about or find out during the next period of time they have together (term, half-term . . .). Explain to the group that this might include how the class will operate, class rules, content or how the class is organised.

b  Allow enough time for each person to finish and then move people into small groups of 3 or 4. Have each group nominate a person to act as recorder. The task is now to make a composite list of objectives and to select priorities.

c  Have the participants discuss what they would like to set as their own priorities. Emphasise that individuals do not have to read out their private lists unless they choose to do so. The recorder notes all the priorities discussed.

d  When the list is complete, ask the group to mark those most mentioned. It is useful to develop a code for topics most mentioned, high priorities, those of lower priority, realistic and unrealistic comments.

e  Bring the small groups back together, and ask a volunteer from each group to read out the list. Develop a list of priorities for the whole group.

f  Use the lists in planning the rest of the course.

g  Keep the lists and refer to them during and at the end of the course as a check that the group is achieving its objectives. Participants keep their own private lists for personal reference during the course.

h  At the end of the course have the group and individuals check what has been achieved against their original objectives and priorities.

# 2 Sentence stems

| | |
|---|---|
| **Objectives** | To gain an immediate reaction from participants about a session. To check that the unit is meeting the participants' expectations. To gain information for further planning. |
| **Prerequisites** | Participation in the session or unit to be evaluated. Literacy skills. |
| **Age group** | 9-13, 13-16, 16 + |
| **Group size** | Any size. |
| **Time needed** | 10-15 minutes. |
| **What you need** | A copy of *Sentence stems* (see examples below), and a pen for each participant. |

**How you do it**

a   Select four appropriate sentence stems and space them on a sheet.

b   Hand out the sentence stems to each participant.

c   Ask each participant to complete the sentences. Explain that these sheets will be handed in and they do not have to sign them. Stress that it is important that they be honest in their responses so that a true picture can be gained.

d   Collect the sheets and collate the responses. If the group is continuing, they may like to see the collated responses.

▶ **Examples of Sentence Stems**

Right now I feel . . .

Next session I hope . . .

The best thing about this session was . . .

One thing I really liked was . . .

I wish I could . . .

I think we could have . . .

I learnt . . .

One thing I didn't like was . . .

I would change . . .

Next time we . . .

This unit has been . . .

# 3 Evaluation voting

**Objectives**      To make a public statement about the session or unit.
                    To move and have fun.
                    To collect information from the group which will assist with future
                    planning.

**Prerequisites**   Participation in the session or unit to be evaluated.

**Age group**       9-13, 13-16, 16 +

**Group size**      Ideally a maximum of 25.

**Time needed**     15 minutes.

**What you need**   Nothing.

**How you do it**

a Explain the hand signals

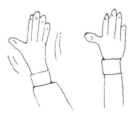 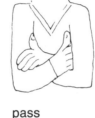 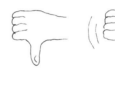

| strongly agree | agree | pass don't know can't decide | disagree | strongly disagree |

b Explain that you will read out a statement (see suggestions below) and
that people should respond quickly with hand signals, not allowing time to
think too much or debate. It is an instant reaction and represents how a
person things right now. At another time their responses may well be
different.

c Read the statements. In this activity it is useful for the educator to
participate also, but delay your voting slightly, because it is possible for
you to influence group members.

▶ **Suggested statements**
I enjoyed the session.
I felt comfortable and relaxed.
I would like to have more discussion on the subject.
I would like to move on to a different subject.
I believe that contraceptive information should be presented in school
courses.
I should like to know more about sexually transmitted diseases.

**Note**            These are a few examples of statements. Design statements to find out
                    what you want to know, either about how the class has progressed
                    generally or about content and subject matter.

# 4 Evaluation ranking

| | |
|---|---|
| **Objectives** | To get feedback from the group about how the course is going. To evaluate material that has been covered, and gain material for future planning. |
| **Prerequisites** | Participation in the course. |
| **Age group** | 13-16, 16 + |
| **Group size** | Any size. |
| **Time needed** | 10-15 minutes. |
| **What you need** | A copy of the statements (see examples below) for each person. |

**How you do it**

a Explain that you would like to find out how the participants feel about the session or course so far. They may or may not wish to sign their evaluation. Participants can be more honest if anonymity is made optional.

b Hand out the evaluation ranking statements, and ask the participants to rank from highest to lowest the statements that best describe their feelings and reactions.

c Explain that it may be difficult to make choices, but that they must make decisions about the order.

d When all are finished, ask the participants to hand in their completed sheets.

▶ **Suggested statements for ranking**
I feel satisfied.
I learnt nothing new.
I wish the other students would be more serious.
I would like more information.
This course is boring.
This course was really great.

**Note**

You can design statements to find out what you want to know, but be certain to balance negative and positive statements.

# 5 Evaluation - field of words

**Objective**                 To find out how the group members are feeling about the session or unit.

**Prerequisites**             Participation in the session or unit to be evaluated.

**Age group**                 13-16, 16 +
                              This activity could be adapted for 9-13 year olds.

**Group size**                Any size.

**Time needed**               15-20 minutes.

**What you need**             A *Field of words* sheet (page 38) for each participant.

**How you do it**

    a  Explain that you will hand out a sheet with words written on it that describe feelings and reactions. Participants can be more honest if anonymity is made optional.

    b  Ask the participants to circle the words that best describe their feelings about the session or unit. They can add their own words if they can't find suitable words on the sheet.

    c  Collect the sheets when they are completed.

# Field of words

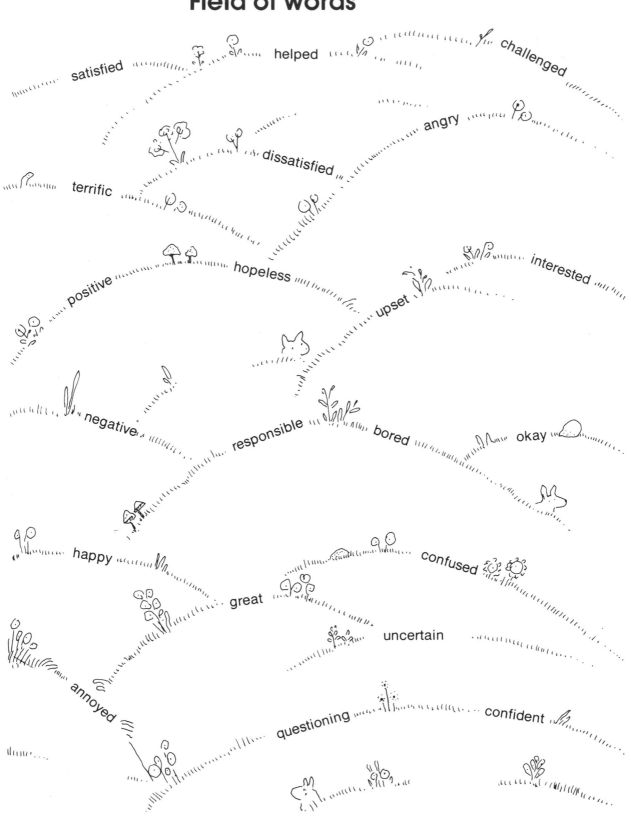

satisfied

helped

challenged

angry

dissatisfied

terrific

hopeless

interested

positive

upset

negative

responsible

bored

okay

happy

confused

great

uncertain

annoyed

questioning

confident

# 6 Review sheets

| | |
|---|---|
| **Objective** | To evaluate a session or unit. |
| **Prerequisites** | Participation in the session or unit to be evaluated. |
| **Age group** | 13-16, 16 + |
| **Group size** | Any size. |
| **Time needed** | 10 minutes. |
| **What you need** | A copy of the appropriate review sheets (pages 40 and 41) for each participant. |

**How you do it**

a Hand out one copy of the review sheet to each person. Participants can be more honest if anonymity is made optional.

b Ask the participants to mark with a cross the point on the continuum that best describes their reactions. Explain that this is to give you an idea of how the course or session went, and how they, as participants felt.

c When they are finished, collect the sheets.

**Note** To evaluate a session, use Form A.
To evaluate a unit, use Form B.

# Form A  Review sheet for the end of a session

Mark an X on the continuum at the point that best describes your reaction.

How satisfied are you with this session?

_____

not satisfied                                                                                    very satisfied

_____

boring?                                                                                              interesting?

COMMENTS
What issues, questions or concerns would you like to include in the next session?

Permission to copy this page for participant use.

# Form B   Review sheet for the end of a unit

Place an X on the continuum at the point which best represents group interest.

_____

0%                                      50%                                      100%

Place an X on the continuum at the point which best represents your participation.

_____

couldn't be bothered                                                      tried my best

Place an X on the continuum which best represents your personal learning.

_____

I learned nothing                                                      I learned a great deal

If I had to give myself a mark for overall participation I think my mark should be

_____

0                25                50                75                100

COMMENTS
If I were planning a unit I would include

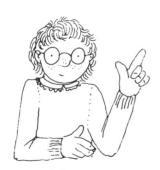

# 7 Telemessages

| | |
|---|---|
| **Objectives** | To ascertain the current issues, concerns and feelings in the group. |
| | To allow the group to share ideals and hopes. |
| | To allow participants to publicly affirm a position on an issue of concern. |
| **Prerequisites** | Literacy skills. |
| **Age group** | 13-16, 16 + |
| **Group size** | Ideally a maximum of 25. |
| **Time needed** | 20-30 minutes. |
| **What you need** | Pens and paper. |

**How you do it**

a Ask participants to think about any one person or group to whom they would like to send a telemessage regarding an issue arising from the sex education course. The telemessage should express how they *feel*, *action* that should be taken, or *policy* that could be developed regarding the issue.

b Allow 5-10 minutes for writing.

c Ask participants if they would like to read their telemessages to the group. State that people need only contribute if they wish to do so.

d The group may like to actually send one of the telemessages. This can be discussed and carried through.

**Note**      This activity can be used for a range of topics.

# 8 Evaluation collage

**Objectives**    To elicit feedback from the participants on their reactions to the unit.
To draw the group together and provide a positive focus to conclude the unit.

**Prerequisites**    Participation in the unit to be evaluated.

**Age group**    9-13, 13-16, 16 +

**Group size**    Ideally a maximum of 25.

**Time needed**    20-30 minutes.

**What you need**    Large sheets of paper, magazines, glue, scissors, display area.

**How you do it**

a Ask the participants to work in small groups.

b Each group is to make a collage, with pictures from the magazines that will depict what the unit meant to them.

c The collages are then displayed and each group explains to the large group what their collages mean.

**Variation**    Instead of pictures, the group may use words and symbols to indicate how they felt about the unit.

# Communicating

In this section of the book, we are presenting activities about building and developing relationships within the group, rather than information about how to communicate. We see developing relationships and effective ways for a group to work together as essential for sex education.

While all the activities in this section could be used in a course or unit on communications, this section is not about teaching communications, but is about developing the process of communicating within the group. To develop a better understanding of the theory and techniques of communication you will find suggested reading on page 46. It is most effective to spread the activities over a period of time, using them both as ice-breakers early in the life of the group progresses. There are two aspects of working in a group that must be built and maintained. The first is the process of the group developing relationships and learning to work together; the second is the task or content. In this section we pay attention to the former, which are the building blocks for achieving the latter. Once a group has established effective patterns of relating the content and task become almost automatic, with group members taking responsibility for their own learning. The educator's role will increasingly become that of a resource person.

The Communicating section is divided into three parts.

1  Introductions.

2  Building and Maintaining Positive Support.

3  Developing Skills in Communicating.

Part 1 deals with getting to know each other. Activities 9-12 are for use early in the life of the group.

Parts 2 and 3 can be used at any stage during the group's time together, but particularly when energy is low, morale is sagging, or the group needs a refreshing burst.

### Factors to consider

Verbal communication (including tone of voice, pitch, the speed of speech and intonation); non-verbal communication (including gestures, eye contact, posture, distance — physical, and breathing rate and rhythm); listening — active and attentive; co-operation versus competition; consensus building; team building; aids and barriers to communication; methods and varieties of communication.

# Communicating

## References
Barnes, D. and Todd, F., *Communication and Learning in Small Groups* Routledge & Kegan Paul, 1977

Brandes, D. and Phillips, H., *Gamesters Handbook*, Hutchinson, 1977

Brandes, D., *Gamesters 2*, Hutchinson, 1982

Ruddock, J., *Learning through Small Group Discussions*, Society for Research into Higher Education, NFER, 1979

Spender, D., *Man Made Language*, Routledge & Kegan Paul, 1980

## Videos/Films
Developmental Work with Tutorial Groups
For Better For Worse
Let's Talk About It
Peege
Why Is It For Them . . . and Not Me?

## Additional Resources
Childhood
Family Lifestyles
Health Education, 13-18: You in a Group, Health and Self
Lifeskills Teaching Programmes, No. 1, No. 2, No. 4

## Activities
Part 1    Introductions

 9  Name game
10  Introducing me
11  'I'd like to introduce you to . . .'
12  Personal collage


Part 2  Building and Maintaining Positive Support

13  Human knots
14  Sitting down circle
15  Building a machine
16  Priorities for life
17  A gift for you


Part 3    Developing Skills in Communicating

18  Aids and barriers to communication
19  Communicating non-verbally
20  Rumours
21  Active listening
22  Observing communication
23  Sexism brainstorm
24  A look at language

# 9 Name game

| | |
|---|---|
| **Objectives** | To reduce nervousness in a new group.<br>To get to know each other.<br>To learn each other's names.<br>To have fun. |
| **Prerequisites** | None. |
| **Age group** | 9-13, 13-16, 16 + |
| **Group size** | Ideally a maximum of 25. |
| **Time needed** | 10-20 minutes, depending on the size of the group. |
| **What you need** | A quiet area large enough for the group to sit in a circle. |

**How you do it**

a  Have the group sit in a circle.

b  Introduce the activity by saying that this is an opportunity to have fun and not a test that can be failed. Participants can be prompted by the rest of the group if they cannot remember.

c  The person to start introduces herself.
Example: 'My name is Mary'.
The next person introduces the person before and then himself.
Example: 'This is Mary and I am Bill'.
The third person names the previous two and then introduces herself and so on, until the entire circle has been introduced.

**Variation**  Add other facts to the name —
a favourite fruit, a word that rhymes with the participant's first name, an adjective that starts with the same letter as the name.
Example: Happy Helen.

**Note**  It is useful for the educator to be last in order to remember everyone's name.

# 10 Introducing me

| | |
|---|---|
| **Objectives** | To get to know each other.<br>To break the ice. |
| **Prerequisites** | Literacy skills. |
| **Age group** | 9-13, 13-16, 16 + |
| **Group size** | Any size. |
| **Time needed** | 20-30 minutes. |
| **What you need** | Paper at least 15 cm square, pins, felt-tip pens. |

**How you do it**

a Give paper, pins and a pen to each person.

b In the middle of the paper have the participants write the name by which they like to be called.

c Ask the participants to write in each corner of the paper as you read out the instructions. Be sure to leave enough time between instructions for each person to finish writing.

d Ask them to write
in the top left corner, how they are feeling right now;
in the top right corner, two things they like to do;
in the bottom left corner, a book or film they have read or seen recently;
and in the bottom right corner, where they would rather be right now.

e Have the participants pin their name tags onto their chests. The educator must be a participant in this activity.

f Have everyone stand, move around the room, read each other's tags and discuss what is written on them. If people seem to be staying with the same person, encourage them to move on so that they may meet as many people as possible.

g Finish discussions when you think everyone has had enough time.

**Follow-up**

This activity can be followed by *'I'd Like to Introduce You to . . .'* (page 49).

**Variation**

You may think of many variations to write around the name tag. A variation we have had fun using is asking the participants to write two things that are true about themselves and one that is false. People then mill around and try to guess which are true and which are false.

# 11 'I'd like to introduce you to . . .'

| | |
|---|---|
| **Objectives** | To get to know each other.<br>To develop listening skills. |
| **Prerequisites** | None. |
| **Age group** | 9-13, 13-16, 16 + |
| **Group size** | Ideally a maximum of 25. |
| **Time needed** | 20-45 minutes. |
| **What you need** | A large comfortable room or area. |

**How you do it**

a  Have the group form into pairs.

b  Explain that the first person in each pair spends about 5 minutes talking about herself or himself. The listener may ask questions to draw out information, but essentially it is that person's job to listen and learn as much as possible about the speaker.

c  After the time is up, call for the pairs to switch roles, and repeat step b.

d  After another five minutes, ask the group to re-form and sit in a circle.

e  Participants in turn introduce their partners, sharing what they have learned from their discussions, until everyone in the group has been introduced.

**Note**

If the introductions from this activity are to follow *Introducing me* (page 48), the name tags can be used as the basis for the discussion in pairs.

With some groups it may be useful to brainstorm the sorts of things they might like to share about themselves.

# 12 Personal collage

| | |
|---|---|
| **Objectives** | To share something of oneself, as a means of introduction.<br>To encourage creative expression.<br>To practise a visual rather than verbal mode of communication. |
| **Prerequisites** | None. |
| **Age group** | 9-13, 13-16, 16 + |
| **Group size** | Ideally a maximum of 25. |
| **Time needed** | 30-45 minutes. |
| **What you need** | Large sheets of paper, glue, scissors, sticky tape, access to the outside environment. |

**How you do it**

a Explain to the participants that they are going to introduce themselves by creating personal collages. The collages should be abstract, and portray some aspects of themselves that they would like to share.

b Allow 15-20 minutes for group members to wander outside collecting seed pods, leaves, twigs or whatever takes their fancy — without destroying the environment.

c Ask the participants to assemble their collages.

d When they are finished, have the participants take turns to explain their portrayals.

**Note**  As this is a personal expression, encourage other group members to listen and not to probe too deeply as there may be some things that a person does not want to share.

# 13 Human knots

| | |
|---|---|
| **Objectives** | To have fun.<br>To provide an opportunity for physical activity.<br>To build trust and acceptance. |
| **Prerequisites** | None. |
| **Age group** | 9-13, 13-16, 16 + |
| **Group size** | Minimum 7, maximum 9 in each small group.<br>Small groups must be uneven numbers. |
| **Time needed** | 15-20 minutes. |
| **What you need** | A large clear space. |

**How you do it**

a If working with a large group, divide into smaller groups with a minimum of seven and have each group stand in a circle facing the centre.

b Everyone crosses their wrists with their arms extended and grasps the hands of two other people opposite them. No individual should be holding both hands of the same person.

c Without letting go of hands, the group then disentangles itself, resulting in an untangled circle with arms uncrossed but still holding hands.

**Variation**

1 Two volunteers leave the room.

2 The group then joins hands, and weaves itself into an impossible knot without breaking any of the connections.

3 The volunteers return and try to direct the untangling of the knot without disconnecting any of the hands.

**Note**

Both of these can be done without any verbal communication, followed by discussion about the ways in which people communicated.

# 14 Sitting down circle

| | |
|---|---|
| **Objectives** | To have fun.<br>To provide an opportunity for physical activity and contact.<br>To build trust and acceptance. |
| **Prerequisites** | None. |
| **Age group** | 9-13, 13-16, 16 + |
| **Group size** | Ideally a maximum of 25. |
| **Time needed** | 15 minutes. |
| **What you need** | A large clear space. |

**How you do it**

a  Have the group stand in a circle, front to back as in an aeroplane. The knees and feet should be touching, and the toes of the person at the back should touch the heels of the person in front.

b  When everyone is tucked up tightly, have them take two small side steps towards the centre.

c  Have the members of the group count 1, 2, 3, and gradually bend their knees to sit down on the knees of the person behind, so that the entire circle is sitting down this way.

d  If it doesn't work at first, try again. When the sitting part is achieved, move on to the hard part where the entire circle walks around in the sitting position.

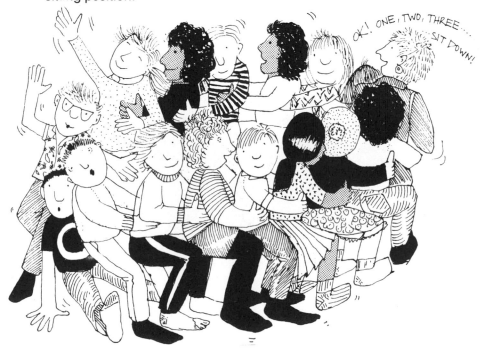

# 15 Building a machine

| | |
|---|---|
| **Objectives** | To have fun.<br>To provide an opportunity for physical movement.<br>To build trust and acceptance. |
| **Prerequisites** | None. |
| **Age group** | 9-13, 13-16, 16 + |
| **Group size** | Any size. |
| **Time needed** | 5-10 minutes. |
| **What you need** | A clear space, large enough to allow movement. |

**How you do it**

a  Explain to the participants that they are going to use their bodies to build an imaginary machine.

b  One person starts a mechanical action, then others attach themselves until a large machine has been built. Each part of the machine should have a specific purpose that can be explained and that contributes to the overall machine.

c  It may help to be more specific and give instructions about what the machine can do.
Example: Let's build a musical machine or a giggle machine.

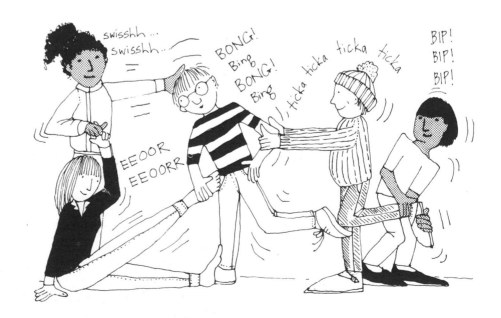

# 16 Priorities for life

| | |
|---|---|
| **Objectives** | To provide participants with an opportunity to see what they prize in their lives.<br>To provide an opportunity to look at past achievements.<br>To allow participants the opportunity to discuss ways of achieving their priorities in the future. |
| **Prerequisites** | Positive support in the group. |
| **Age group** | 9-13, 13-16, 16+ |
| **Group size** | Ideally a maximum of 25. |
| **Time needed** | 30-45 minutes. |
| **What you need** | Paper, pens. |

**How you do it**

a Hand out paper and pens.

b Explain the objectives of the activity.

c Have each person draw a line across the page.

d Tell the participants to write the year of their birth at the beginning of the line. At the end of the line they write the year of their projected demise. They can decide now at what age they want to die! They then mark on the line their present age and the current year. Every person now has a line representing their past, present and future.

e Between their birth and the present, the participants mark in what they see as significant events in their lives to date. Between the present and their death, they write down the things they would like to achieve in the future. These may be personal or public accomplishments, big or small.

f Ask them to look at the side of the page that represents the future and note how they feel about that list.
Is it realistic?
Can any be achieved in the forseeable future?
What will they have to do to achieve it?

**Follow-up**
This activity may be followed by *Setting objectives and priorities* (page 33) or by *Promises to myself* (page 74) to start action on one of the priorities.

# 17 A gift for you

| | |
|---|---|
| **Objectives** | To improve the self-image of group members.<br>To consolidate feelings of positive support within the group.<br>To provide an opportunity for group members to express positive farewells at the end of a course. |
| **Prerequisites** | Positive support in the group. |
| **Age group** | 9-13, 13-16, 16 + |
| **Group size** | Ideally a maximum of 25. |
| **Time needed** | 30-45 minutes. |
| **What you need** | Small pieces of paper, pens, one large clearly named envelope for each participant. |

**How you do it**

a Hand out small pieces of paper so that each person has one piece for every other member of the group.

b Each person writes an individual message to each other person in the group. The messages must be positive and may refer to physical or personality traits.

c Fold each message, and on it write the name of the person it is meant for. Messages may be signed or unsigned as a matter of personal preference.

d While the messages are being written, arrange the named envelopes as letterboxes.

e Have the participants deliver the messages into the letterboxes.

f Participants then pick up their post and read their messages. Allow time for the group members to share how they feel about their messages and the activity itself.

**Note** The educator should be a participant in this activity.

# A gift for you

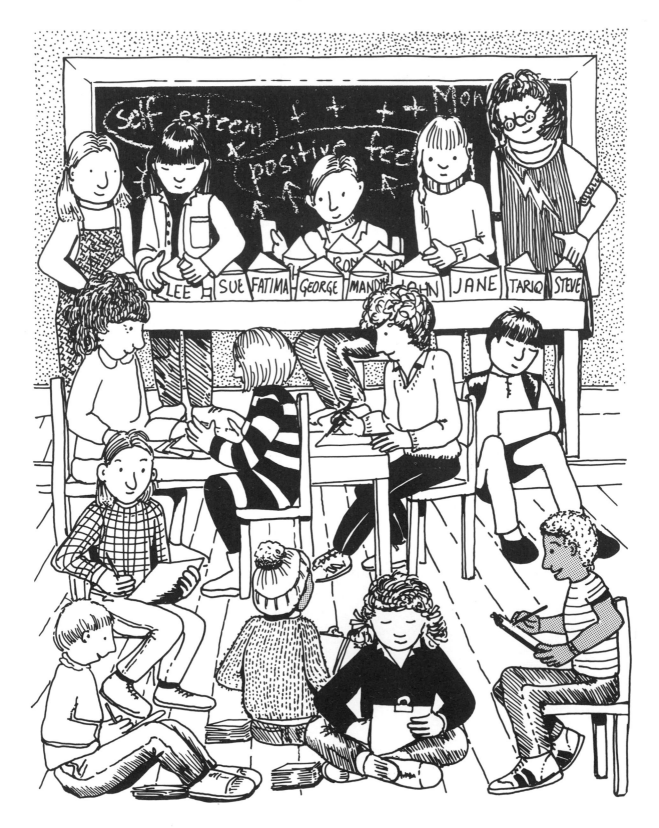

# **18** Aids and barriers to communication

| | |
|---|---|
| **Objectives** | To assist participants to identify the barriers or problems in inter-personal communication.<br>To promote an understanding of effective communication.<br>To discuss the skills of communicating.<br>To help identify specific areas for further work. |
| **Prerequisites** | A common understanding of interpersonal communication. |
| **Age group** | 13-16, 16 + |
| **Group size** | Ideally a maximum of 25. |
| **Time needed** | 45 minutes. |
| **What you need** | Paper, felt-tip pens. |

**How you do it**

a  Divide the group into small groups.

b  Instruct the small groups to find a working space where they can talk and write comfortably.

c  Explain that without discussing each point, they are to list all the barriers to communication — things that make communicating difficult.
Allow 5-10 minutes.

d  On another piece of paper they are to list all the aids to communication — those things that make communicating easier.
Allow 5-10 minutes.

e  Allow time for each group to discuss its list and clarify the points made.

f  Ask each group to share its list and form a composite list.

g  Ask individuals or groups to identify areas which they would like to pursue through further discussion or practical activities.

# 19 Communicating non-verbally

| | |
|---|---|
| **Objectives** | To demonstrate that people are communicating even when they are not using words.<br>To increase awareness of non-verbal behaviours. |
| **Prerequisites** | None. |
| **Age group** | 9-13, 13-16, 16 + |
| **Group size** | Any size. |
| **Time needed** | 20-30 minutes. |
| **What you need** | A comfortable working space. |

**How you do it**

a Each participant selects a partner and they find a working space.

b The partners face each other either sitting or standing.

c Participants take turns to choose an attitude or emotion, and without words communicate this to their partner.

d Allow time for discussion about how the emotions were conveyed and how they were interpreted.

**Variations**

1 Without talking, have one partner mould the other into a position to demonstrate an emotion or attitude. Either the moulded person or the whole group guesses the emotion or attitude portrayed.

2 Hand each person a sealed envelope containing a written instruction to act to the total group. Members of the group guess the emotion or attitude being communicated.

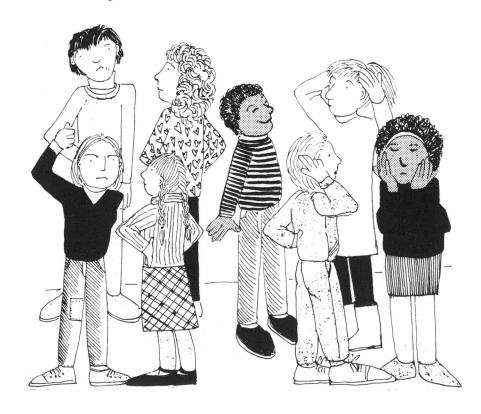

# **20** Rumours

| | |
|---|---|
| **Objectives** | To examine the ways in which messages are often distorted.<br>To introduce participants to listening skills.<br>To demonstrate the problems of one way communication. |
| **Prerequisites** | None. |
| **Age group** | 13-16, 16 + |
| **Group size** | Ideally a maximum of 25. |
| **Time needed** | 35-45 minutes. |
| **What you need** | A written message of no more than 75 words. The message should be of relevance and interest to the group. |

**How you do it**

a  Ask for 5 volunteers to leave the room. The rest of the participants act as observers.

b  Explain to the five volunteers that they will be recalled one at a time to receive a verbal message, which is to be passed on to the next volunteer. The message will be stated once only to each person.

c  Call the first person back into the room. The educator reads the message aloud (see examples below). It is then passed on from memory. The second person is called into the room and hears the message from the first person. Repeat the process until the fifth person receives the message from the fourth person. The fifth person repeats the message to the total group.

d  The educator re-reads the original message, and the distortions, deletions and mistakes are noted.

e  Allow time for the five volunteers to discuss how they felt and what happened to them during the process.

f  Total group discussion can focus on how and why the message became distorted.

**Note**

Recorders can be appointed from the group to note on paper the distortions, deletions and mistakes as they occur.

▶ **Examples of messages for rumours**

So glad I caught you, the Head has just told Pat that each house is to elect four representatives to work with the School Council on the planning for the school fete and disco. Each house is to organise a meeting tomorrow and have elections so that the reps can meet on Thursday and send their ideas to the Council Meeting on Monday. Can you organise your house for a meeting tomorrow? Thanks a lot.

Hey, I've been trying to find you. John can't come to the disco tomorrow at Riverside. He's got to go out with his mum. Can you ask Paula if Andrew would like John's ticket. If so, will he meet John by the main school entrance at four o'clock. If not, let me know on the bus tonight, because my brother might want to come. The disco starts at 7pm, and the ticket costs £1.50 (food included).

# **21** Active listening

| | |
|---|---|
| **Objectives** | To explore the importance of active listening. |
| | To provide participants with practice in listening. |
| | To increase listening skills. |
| **Prerequisites** | An introduction to communication by an activity such as *Aids and barriers to communication* (page 57). |
| **Age group** | 13-16, 16 + |
| **Group size** | Any size. |
| **Time needed** | 20-30 minutes. |
| **What you need** | A list of possible issues (see suggestions below). |

**How you do it**

a  Each participant chooses a partner and they find a working space.

b  The issue to be discussed is selected from the list.

c  Ask one of the pair to be the speaker and the other the listener.

d  Explain that after the speaker has made a statement on the issue, the listener must repeat the substance of the statement to the speaker's satisfaction before another point is introduced.

e  After 4 minutes, change roles.

f  After another 4 minutes, allow the pairs to discuss the activity, noting what they learnt about the difficulties of listening and what was good about being listened to.

g  Share the experience with the large group.

▶ **Suggested active listening issues**

Women and men should take equal roles in raising children.

Marriages are made in heaven.

Sex without love is hollow.

Sex education should be an integral part of every school curriculum.

Sexual experience is best gained within marriage.

Men should take more responsibility for birth control.

AIDS should be an issue of concern to all of us.

# 22 Observing communication

| | |
|---|---|
| **Objective** | To increase awareness about the range of ways in which we communicate. |
| **Prerequisites** | An understanding of the concepts involved in verbal and non-verbal communication. |
| **Age group** | 16 + |
| **Group size** | Minimum of 10, maximum of 25. |
| **Time needed** | 30-45 minutes. |
| **What you need** | Paper, pens. |

**How you do it**

a The educator and another person prepare a 3 to 5 minute role-play (page 23), prior to the session. This involves one person taking the role of the initiator, the other of the respondant in a dialogue. The initiator starts a pre-decided conversation of mutual interest and displays a range of behaviours during the conversation.
Example: interest, lack of interest, boredom, agitation, and excitement. The respondant participates by trying to maintain communication in spite of the behaviour of the initiator. This role-play does not have to be rehearsed, only prepared.

b Prior to commencement of the role-play, each member of the group is assigned a verbal or non-verbal behaviour to observe.
These should include:
the words used
eye movement
gestures
posture
tone of voice
eye contact
body position
breathing
blushing
paling
sweating

c At the end of the role-play both players must derole.

d Ask the observers to report what they saw, and how it affected the interaction. Discuss the importance of verbal and non-verbal messages and how these apply to everyday communication.

**Note**  Topics for the conversation could include the work they do, films they have enjoyed, the economic crisis, important relationships, or holidays.

# 23 Sexism brainstorm

| | |
|---|---|
| **Objectives** | To highlight sexism in our language.<br>To introduce participants to the concept of sex role stereotypes. |
| **Prerequisites** | None. |
| **Age group** | 13-16, 16 +<br>This activity could be adapted for 9-13 year olds. |
| **Group size** | Ideally a maximum of 25. |
| **Time needed** | 20-30 minutes. |
| **What you need** | Large sheets of paper, felt-tip pens, dictionary and thesaurus. |
| **How you do it** | |

a Have the group divide into 8 groups of equal size and find working spaces. Give each group a piece of paper and felt-tip pen, and ask them to nominate a recorder.

b Assign one of the following words to each group and ask the recorder to write it on the top of the page.

| | |
|---|---|
| male | lady |
| female | gentleman |
| man | weak |
| woman | strong |

c Outline the rules for brainstorming (page 21).
Have each group brainstorm all the words and phrases that are associated with their word.

d In the large group, compare the list of words and discuss the similarities and differences. It may be useful to add to the lists with synonyms from a thesaurus.

e Focus the discussion on words and phrases that stereotype female and male behaviour. Have the group work towards formulating a definition of sexism and sex role stereotypes.

| | |
|---|---|
| **Follow-up** | In small groups, discuss and note the effect the attitudes expressed in their lists have on them as females and males. |
| **Note** | Omit some of the words if the group is not large enough to form 8 small groups. |

# **24** A look at language

| | |
|---|---|
| **Objectives** | To increase awareness of the sexism implicit in our language. To assist participants to find alternative non-sexist words and phrases. |
| **Prerequisites** | None. |
| **Age group** | 13-16, 16 + |
| **Group size** | Minimum of 6. |
| **Time needed** | 40-45 minutes. |
| **What you need** | 4 copies of the sketch (page 64), paper, pen, and a copy of *A look at language — reference sheet* (page 65), for each participant. |

**How you do it**

a The educator finds four volunteers willing to perform the sketch. These can be female or male, but the roles remain masculine. Each is given a copy of the dialogue and sent away for 10 minutes to prepare.

b During this time, explain to the remainder of the participants that they are to act as observers while the sketch is being performed. They are to write down any sexist or discriminatory words or phrases in the dialogue.

c At the conclusion of the sketch, allow the observers time to finish their notes.

d Re-enact the sketch allowing the observers to interject at the points that they think are sexist or discriminatory. Explore each one as it arises, encouraging discussion of alternatives.

e Hand out a copy of *A look at language — reference sheet* to each participant for personal reference.

**Follow-up**

1 Ask the participants to write a similar sketch which is non-sexist.

2 *Re-sexing the ads* (page 90).

**Variation**

The sketch can be performed with young women reading both the parts and changing all the masculine references to feminine.
Example: 'Hi Veena, Sue, Vicky — how's the mister?'

# A look at language

**Scene: Party one Saturday night**
A group of people are standing around eating and drinking.

Bill: Hi Winston, hello, Gary — how's the missus?

Gary: She's over there with the kids of course. She's been a bit uppity since getting a job, earning her own pin money.

Bill: Yeah, I know what you mean, my missus thinks she can get her GCSE's if she goes back to college. I've told her there's no chance, not if she tries Maths and Science anyway. Would you believe it, she wants to be a woman engineer.

Help yourself to drinks.

Gary: Want another pint, Bill?

Bill: Yeah, thanks.

Pete: What about the birds?

Bill: Ah, don't worry about them, they're busy in the kitchen. Wait till they've finished there or we'll never get anything to eat — you know women.

Winston: What's your wife's little sideline then, Gary?

Gary: She's a postman.

Bill: OK kids, go and play. You girls can play with the dolls house upstairs in the bedroom. You boys take a football and go out in the street for a kick — watch the traffic though. Why don't we sit down?

Pete: Hey, mind the cat, Winston. Poor old fella he only wants an easy life.

Winston: This chair's a bit wobbly. You should fix it Bill.

Bill: Yeah, I know, you're right. My wife's been nagging me for weeks to fix it.

Gary: It's great having a chance to relax. Oh good, the ladies are producing the food — let's eat.

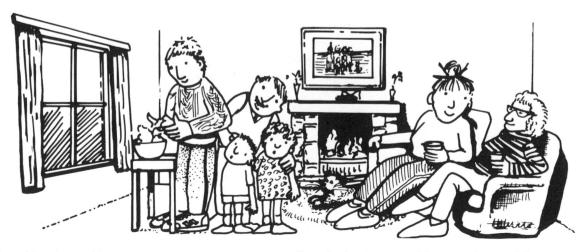

# A look at language - reference sheet

| | |
|---|---|
| 'the missus' | Denotes marriage. Women tend to be referred to by their marital status, men are not. Women usually take their father's name at birth, and their husband's name when they marry. There is no legal requirement for this. Ms. is an acceptable alternative.<br>Also objectifies a woman — she doesn't have a name. |
| 'with the kids of course' | Implies that women should be with the children as a matter of course. |
| 'She's been a bit uppity' | 'Uppity' is a word sometimes used for women who try to step into positions that are traditionally seen as male roles. |
| 'pin money' | Assumption that the money earned is extra, and not a valuable contribution to the family budget. |
| 'thinks she can get her GCSE's — no chance — Maths and Science' | Women are often belittled for trying anything intellectual, academic technical or scientific. |
| 'woman engineer' | Why 'woman'? We don't specify 'man engineer'. |
| 'birds' | A derogatory term for women, objectifying them and grouping them all together as pretty, cute and brainless. Throughout the scene women are never referred to by their names. |
| 'they're busy in the kitchen' | Assumes that women will automatically be found in the kitchen preparing food. |
| 'you know women' | Is a generalisation of women's behaviour, implying that all women behave in a certain way and that it is understood that they do. |
| 'little sideline' | Again a belittling of a woman's role as a contributor to the family income, and an assumption that her work outside the home is less important than that within. |
| 'postman' | Why do we go on using male terminology? Postwoman, post person, post officer or letter carrier would be alternative terms. They may sound strange at first, but nobody thinks baker, butcher, carpenter and builder should be bakeman, butchman, carpentman or buildman. |
| 'girls — dolls house' 'boys — football' | Certain playthings have become traditionally female or male. Why shouldn't all children be encouraged to play with a range of toys? |
| 'in the bedroom' 'in the street' | Girls are often protected, whilst boys are allowed the freedom to explore. All children need both at different times. |
| 'poor old fella, he' | If in doubt about the sex of an animal it tends to be assumed that it is male. This implies that the natural state of affairs in our society is masculine: therefore normal equals masculine. He, his and him are used to describe everything from wild animals and birds, whose sex we don't know, to mixed crowds of women and men whose sex we do know. |
| 'you should fix it Bill' | Men are traditionally seen as practical, but they are not necessarily comfortable in this role. Women generally are not expected to know how to fix things. |
| 'I know, you're right. My wife's been nagging . . .' | The point is agreed with when a man makes it, but it is regarded as nagging when made by a woman. Classifying a statement as nagging diminishes both the problem and the person. |
| 'the ladies' | Puts women into a particular category again, and labels their role, rather than recognising them as individuals. |

Permission to copy this page for participant use.

# Relationships

## Factors to Consider

Self-esteem, communication, expectations, feelings, attitudes, needs diversity, sex roles, sexism, socialisation, responsibility, exploitations, power, stages.

## Words the Educator May Want to Know and Understand

Friendship, sexual, platonic, peers, lover, parents, child, student, teacher, living together, de facto, family, marriage, contract, short term, lifelong, divorce, love, caring, sharing, destructive, painful, manipulating, forming, maintaining, ending, celibate, heterosexual, homosexual, lesbian, bisexual, monogamy, non-monogamy, polyandry, polygamy, polgyny, serial monogamy.

## References

Brown, P. and Faulder, C., *Treat Yourself to Sex: A Guide to Good Loving*, Penguin, 1979
Canfield, J. and Wells, H., *100 Ways to Enhance Self-Concept in the Classroom,* Prentice Hall Inc., New Jersey, 1976
Hart, J. and Richardson, D., *The Theory and Practice of Homosexuality*, Routledge & Kegan Paul, 1981
Hemming, S., (ed), *Girls are Powerful*, Sheba Feminist Publishers, 1982
Simon, S., et al, *Values Clarification*, Hart Publishing Co., Inc., New York, 1972
Trenchard, L., (ed), *Talking About Young Lesbians*, London Gay Teenage Group, 1984
Warren, H., *Talking About School*, London Gay Teenage Group, 1984
Warren, H. and Trenchard, L., *Something to Tell You*, London Gay Teenage Group, 1984

## Reading for Participants

Adams, C. and Laurikietis, R., *The Gender Trap: A Closer Look at Sex Roles — Messages and Images*, Virago, 1976
Claesson, B. H., *Boy, Girl, Man, Woman: A Guide to Sex for Young People*, Penguin, 1980
(This book was written for young people, but some educators may prefer to use it for reference only.)
Cousins, J., *Make It Happy*, Penguin, 1979
(This book was written for young people, but some educators may prefer to use it for reference only.)
Hart, J., *So You Think You're Attracted to the Same Sex?* Penguin, 1984
Heron, A., (ed), *One Teenager in Ten*, Alyson Publications Inc., Boston, 1983
Rayner, C., *Growing Pains — and How To Avoid Them*, Corgi, 1984
Note: This list does not include fiction for teenagers. There are many books which raise issues about relationships.

## Videos/Films

For Better for Worse
Framed Youth — Revenge of the Teenage Perverts
Girls Talk
Give Us A Smile
Gregory's Girl
Homosexuality — What About McBride?
The Impossible Dream
I, Myself series: Sean and Joel
I, Myself series: Tracy and Trevor
Learning to Love

**Relationships**

Like Other People
Loving and Caring
Peege
Somebody's Daughter
Starting Point Films: Thinking About Conflict
True Romance etc.
Us Girls
Why Is It For Them . . . And Not Me?

**Additional resources**

All Right for Some
Changing Images
Childhood
Discussion Cards
Divorce and Children
Doing things In and About the Home
Fit for Life
Family Lifestyles
Gender Equality
Genderwatch!
Greater Expectations
Health Action Pack
Health Education, 13-18: You in a Group, Health and Self
Health Matters
It's Your Life: Sex Roles
Lifeskills Teaching Programmes No. 1, No. 4
Life (Talking Points, Set 2)
Living Choices
Male and Female (CRAC)
Roles, Relationships, Responsibilities
Sexuality and the Mentally Handicapped: Parts 4, 8
Think Well: Units 1, 2
Understanding Others
What Is a Family?
Who Are You Staring At?

**Activities**

# **25** What is a relationship

| | |
|---|---|
| **Objectives** | To facilitate discussion about relationships and the range of relationships. To reach a common working definition of the term relationship. |
| **Prerequisites** | None. |
| **Age group** | 13-16, 16 + |
| **Group size** | Ideally a maximum of 25. |
| **Time needed** | 45 minutes. |
| **What you need** | Large sheets of paper, felt-tip pens, a large comfortable area. |

**How you do it**

a Divide the group into small groups of 3 or 4.

b Ask each group to nominate a recorder.

c Give one instruction at a time and leave 5 minutes between each instruction. Ask each group to discuss, and the recorder to keep notes, on the following:
What is a relationship?
What types of relationships are there?
What are the components of a positive relationship?
What are the components of a negative relationship?

d When each topic has been discussed, ask the small groups to return to the total group.

e Ask the recorders to report their findings.

f Help the group to identify any similarities and differences between each small group's findings.

g Conduct a general discussion about the points which emerge and agree upon a working definition.

**Variation**  Friendship could be explored in the same way, with questions like:
What is friendship?
How do you know if somebody is a friend?
What do you look for in a friendship?
What are the degrees of friendship?

# **26** Friendship circles

| | |
|---|---|
| **Objectives** | To enable participants to see different levels of friendships.<br>To offer a starting point for developing friendship patterns. |
| **Prerequisites** | Positive support in the group. Some preliminary discussion of friendship, degrees of friendship (see *What is a relationship*, variation, page 69). |
| **Age group** | 13-16, 16 + |
| **Group size** | Ideally a maximum of 25. |
| **Time needed** | 45 minutes. |
| **What you need** | Paper, felt-tip pens. |

**How you do it**

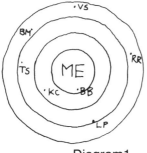

Diagram1

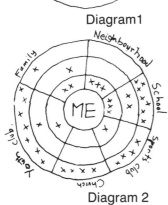

Diagram 2

a State that the content of this activity is private. The patterns that emerge will be different and may change at times for each participant.

b Ask each person to take a sheet of paper and write ME in the centre, then draw four concentric circles around ME (see diagram 1). These circles will represent the degrees of closeness or distance identified in the previous discussion.

c Ask participants to indicate, by using initials or a code, the positions of their friends in the circles.

d Ask participants to look at their diagrams and to think about what they see and how they feel.

e Allow time for discussion. Explore how their friendship patterns may change and how they can be changed.

| | |
|---|---|
| **Follow-up** | Further sessions may be allocated to drawing patterns for the time period two years ago, four years ago, or the projected future 'ideal' circle. |
| **Variations** | |

1 Codes may be used to differentiate between different groups that friends belong to.
Example: female, male, school, home, clubs.
Lines may also be used to connect these groups, some of which may overlap.

2 Following step b, divide the circles into the different segments that participants can identify in their lives.
Example: school, club, home, family, sport.
Place friends in the segments where they belong and indicate their closeness or distance (see diagram 2).

70

# **27** Me and my world

| | |
|---|---|
| **Objectives** | To provide participants with a framework within which to view their relationships.<br>To stimulate discussion about the range of relationships. |
| **Prerequisites** | An atmosphere of trust and acceptance within the group, and with the educator. Some consensus on a definition of relationship.<br>See *What is a relationship?* (page 69). |
| **Age group** | 16+ |
| **Group size** | Ideally a maximum of 25. |
| **Time needed** | 30 minutes to 1 hour. |
| **What you need** | Paper, pens. |

**How you do it**

a State that the content of this activity is private. Participants' feelings about the activity can be shared at the end of the session.

b Provide each person with a sheet of paper and a pen.

c Ask participants to list on the left side of the paper those people who are important to them. The fact that the lists will be different for each person should be made clear, as each will have a different definition of importance.

d Explain that they will draw a diagram to represent how close or distant the people on their lists are in relation to themselves. They start by writing their own names in the centre of the page (see diagram).

e Using names, symbols or initials, ask them to plot the people from their lists to indicate how close or distant they are in proximity to themselves.

f Stress that this is a picture of our relationships today. It may differ tomorrow and probably was different yesterday. Relationships change and develop.

g Ask participants to look at their diagrams and to think about what they see, and how they feel.

h Then ask them to reflect on this and complete one or more of the following sentences:
I discovered that I . . .
It seems that . . .
I was surprised that I . . .

i Provide the opportunity for participants to share anything they would like to about the activity, either in pairs or in the large group.

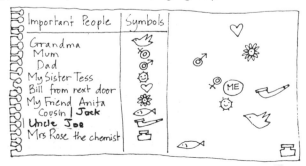

71

# 28 Relationships collage

| | |
|---|---|
| **Objectives** | To enable participants to explore the characteristics of one or more of their important relationships. |
| | To provide an activity whereby participants creatively express their interpretation of their relationships. |
| **Prerequisites** | None. |
| **Age group** | 9-13, 13-16, 16 + |
| **Group size** | Ideally a maximum of 25. |
| **Time needed** | 60-90 minutes. |
| **What you need** | Large sheets of paper, string, glue, sticky tape, scissors, collage materials, access to the external environment. |

**How you do it**

a Ask the participants to close their eyes and think of a relationshp that is or has been important to them. Allow time for thought.

b Ask the participants to create collages portraying those important relationships. This is to be done using the resources available. If possible, have the participants go outside to collect natural objects without damaging the environment.

c When the participants have finished, divide into small groups of 3 or 4 so they may look at each other's collages.

d They may also like to talk about them. This may be general or detailed discussion.

e Display the collages if the participants agree.

# **29** Relationship matrix

**Objectives**    To enable participants to gain a picture of their relationships.
             To assist participants to develop strategies for maintaining or changing
             their relationships.

**Prerequisites**   An atmosphere of positive support within the group. Participation in *What
             is a relationship?* (page 69).

**Age group**    13-16, 16 +

**Group size**    Ideally a maximum of 25.

**Time needed**   45 minutes.

**What you need**  Paper, pens.

**How you do it**

a  State that the content of this activity is private. The participants may say
   how they felt about the activity at the conclusion.

b  Hand each participant a sheet of paper and ask them to draw two lines
   crossing in the centre of the page. The two poles of one line represent
   close and distant. The other two poles are positive and negative.
   Participants may use their own definitions of positive, negative, close and
   distant.

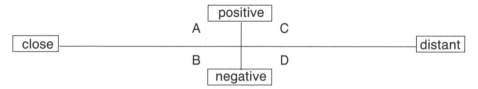

In this diagram, A represents a close and positive, or good relationship;
B, a close and negative relationship. C represents a positive, and distant
relationship; and D a negative and distant relationship.

c  Demonstrate and explain the matrix as shown in the diagram.

d  Ask each person to think about the people with whom they have
   relationships and to mark them where they fit on the page.

e  Allow time for the participants to complete their diagrams. Stress the right
   to confidentiality and state that these are 'photographs' for today and
   may change tomorrow.

f  Ask the participants to look at their diagrams and circle those
   relationships which they would like to change. Then ask them to draw an
   arrow to the position on the diagram where they would like them to be.
   For example, a close negative (B) to a distant negative (D).

g  Ask the participants to individually and privately identify the practical
   actions and initiatives they need to take in order to achieve these
   changes.

h  Provide the opportunity for students to share and practise their strategies
   in either the small group or the total group.

i  Initiate discussion in the group to allow participants to express what they
   think or feel as a result of doing the activity.

**Follow-up**    *Promises to myself* (page 74).

# **30** Promises to myself

**Objectives**    To assist participants to identify areas of their lives that they wish to develop or change.
To encourage participants to work out appropriate ways to achieve these changes.

**Prerequisites**    An indication of interest by individual participants in changing some aspect(s) of their behaviour.

**Age group**    9-13, 13-16. 16 +

**Group size**    Ideally a maximum of 25.

**Time needed**    20-30 minutes.

**What you need**    Nothing.

**How you do it**

a  Ask the participants to think of an aspect in their lives that they would like to change. It could be to start something, to stop something or to change something.

b  Explain the idea that people may want to make a contract in order to promise action towards change. A contract involves agreeing to achieve a certain action in a certain time.

c  Have each person draw up a contract by writing the following:

I ........................................................................................ (name)
promise that by ........................................................... (date)
I will ........................................................... (fill in the promise)
by doing ........................................................... (outline how)
(Signed) ........................................................................................

Let individuals in the group decide whether to keep the content of the contract private. Some participants may want to share their resolutions with others in the group.

d  Agree on the date for checking back and make time on that day for discussion and celebration, or new contract making.

**Note**    This activity is a useful follow-up to any activity dealing with how people live their lives.
Try to keep the contracts achievable and realistic, or the idea may fall flat. Impress on the group that small steps often go further than giant leaps.

# **31** A story in parts

**Objectives**        To explore attitudes to relationships in an enjoyable and creative manner.
To develop communication skills.
To provide a group building activity.
To have fun.

**Prerequisites**      None.

**Age group**        13-16, 16 +
This activity could be adapted for 9-13 year olds.

**Group size**       Ideally a maximum of 25.

**Time needed**     30-45 minutes.

**What you need**   A tape recorder, paper and pens, or blackboard and chalk.

**How you do it**

a  Everyone should sit comfortably in a circle with the tape recorder in the middle.

b  The leader commences a story about a relationship of some kind (see examples below). The story is gradually developed by each person in the group adding two or three sentences consecutively and then passing the story to the next person. Everyone has the right to miss a turn. As characters are introduced write their names in clear view.

c  Stop the story after two or three times around the circle, or when the group chooses.

d  Play back the recorded story. Ask the participants to listen for the attitudes being expressed.

e  List the attitudes expressed. Note the assumptions made about relationships in the way the story developed. Include assumptions about relationships between females and between males.

f  Discuss the factors that influence our attitudes towards relationships.

▶**Examples of commencing statements**

They walked down the path together towards the bench where they had first met . . .

In great distress, Sam rushed out of the house, slamming the door, and ran into the street crying, 'You all hate me, I know'.

They were holding hands as they walked down the street. Mary thought Pat was a special friend.

# 32 Identifying assumptions

| | |
|---|---|
| **Objectives** | To raise and clarify some of the everyday assumptions people make. To identify and discuss some of those assumptions and look at the reasons they are made. |
| **Prerequisites** | None. |
| **Age group** | 13-16, 16 + |
| **Group size** | Ideally a maximum of 25. |
| **Time needed** | 40 minutes. |
| **What you need** | A copy of *Identifying assumptions — the story* and *statements about the story* (page 77) for each person. |

**How you do it**

a Hand out copies of the story and ask group members not to discuss it. Read the story out aloud.

b When the story has been read, ask the participants to circle privately their responses to each statement.

c Then read out each statement and ask the participants to indicate their responses. Have a volunteer from each of the response groupings explain the reason for her or his choice.

d Discuss the assumptions that influenced their choices.

e Repeat this procedure for each statement.

**Follow-up** During the following week, have the group members observe and note common assumptions as they encounter them. These lists can be brought back to a following session for further discussion.

# Identifying assumptions: the story

Viv and Chris walked down the street holding hands. They were very close, and even though they were only sixteen they were sure they loved each other. 'It's not fair, Chris', said Viv, 'your parents give you such an easy time, why don't mine?' Viv's parents were strict, and expected to be obeyed. Viv wanted to finish school and become a nurse, but at times it all seemed too much. It was only Chris's support that kept Viv going.

For Chris things were different. Chris planned to finish school, become an apprentice and work hard to do well. With parents who thought those plans were fine and expected their children to be responsible for their own decisions and lives, Chris felt really lucky.

It was sometimes hard to understand why they felt so attracted to each other, as they came from such different backgrounds.

**Circle your response to each of the following statements:**

| Statements about the story | True | False | Don't know |
|---|---|---|---|
| Viv and Chris plan to become engaged. | T | F | ? |
| Viv is a girl. | T | F | ? |
| Chris is a boy. | T | F | ? |
| Viv does well at school. | T | F | ? |
| Viv and Chris are in love. | T | F | ? |
| Viv and Chris want to live together. | T | F | ? |
| Viv's parents want to keep Viv and Chris apart. | T | F | ? |
| Apprenticeships are for boys. | T | F | ? |
| Nursing is for girls. | T | F | ? |
| Viv and Chris are both girls. | T | F | ? |
| Viv and Chris are both boys. | T | F | ? |

# **33** Homosexuality — interview

| | |
|---|---|
| **Objectives** | To answer questions about homosexuality.<br>To discuss the myths, misconceptions and truths about homosexuality. |
| **Prerequisites** | An atmosphere of positive support and trust. |
| **Age group** | 16 + |
| **Group size** | Ideally a maximum of 25. |
| **Time needed** | At least three sessions. |
| **What you need** | A tape recorder, blank tapes. |
| **How you do it** | |

a You will need to find a co-operative resource person; a lesbian or male homosexual (preferably both) to carry out this project.

b Explain to the group members that they will have an opportunity to ask a lesbian or male homosexual any questions they would like about homosexuality. This will be done by preparing a list of questions and recording them.

c When the tape has been made, send it to the resource person so that she or he can tape the answers and comments, and send them back to the group. In a later session the tape can be played and discussed.

d If appropriate, the resource person can be invited along to a later session as a visiting speaker. Follow the procedure for Visiting speakers (page 25).

| | |
|---|---|
| **Follow-up** | After the project has been completed, a discussion period may be valuable. Focus the discussion on such things as assumptions people make about lesbians and male homosexuals, the attitudes of both individuals and society, and other important issues and points that may emerge. |
| **Note** | Educators may not feel comfortable with the idea of inviting in a lesbian or a male homosexual, and governing bodies of schools may consider it unacceptable. |
| | However, for some young people this can be an effective way of challenging prejudice and increasing tolerance. |
| | You will need to consider carefully the possible outcomes of using this activity. |

# **34** Values frames

| | |
|---|---|
| **Objectives** | To enable private and personal examination of values and attitudes related to sexual preference.<br>To encourage public discussion about sexual preference and the myths and taboos surrounding homosexuality. |
| **Prerequisites** | An atmosphere of positive support and acceptance within the group. |
| **Age group** | 16 + |
| **Group size** | Ideally a maximum of 25. |
| **Time needed** | 30-40 minutes. |
| **What you need** | A sheet of paper and a pen for each person. |

**How you do it**

a Explain that this is essentially a private activity and that while no sharing is required, discussion related to it will occur later.

b Ask the participants to draw a square large enough to contain one word in the centre of their pages. Draw six squares of similar size around the central square.

c Have them write the word 'homosexual' in the centre square and then write the first words that come into their heads in the other squares. Stress that they need not fill in all the squares if they get stuck for words, and that they can write more than six words if they want to.

d Without any discussion, have the participants turn over their paper and prepare the page as before. This time in the centre square, they should write the word 'heterosexual', and then all the words that come to mind in the other squares.

e Now ask the participants to look on both sides of their paper at the kind of words they have written. Ask if these words give any consistent picture about their attitudes or feelings. Ask them to check the words that are the same on both sides of the paper and then select the word that best describes their reaction to each topic.

f To draw all this information together, ask the participants to complete one of the *Sentence stems* (page 34).

g Discussion could then focus on attitudes:
Where do our attitudes come from?
How do we learn them?
Why are there taboos surrounding homosexuality in our society?
Are they changing?

# 35 My parents

| | |
|---|---|
| **Objective** | To facilitate discussion on relationships between young people and their parents. |
| **Prerequisites** | An understanding of effective communication skills. |
| **Age group** | 13-16, 16 +<br>This activity could be adapted for 9-13 year olds, using different pictures. |
| **Group size** | Ideally a maximum of 25. |
| **Time needed** | 30-40 minutes. |
| **What you need** | A copy of the cartoons (page 81) and a pen for each participant. |

**How you do it**

a  Hand out copies of the cartoons.

b  Ask each participant to make up the dialogue for the empty bubbles.

c  Allow 15-20 minutes for everyone to complete the cartoons.

d  Focus discussion on what participants write in the bubbles.

▶ **Suggested discussion topics**

What are the important factors for effective communication with parents?

Why do parents try to control and discipline their children's lives?

Do parents have different expectations for girls and boys?

What are some ways for young people to enable their parents to understand their point of view?

| | |
|---|---|
| **Variation** | These cartoon situations and their outcomes may be role-played instead of completing the dialogue bubbles. |
| **Note** | Educators need to be sensitive to the home situation of participants. Not all of them will be living with parents. |

# My parents

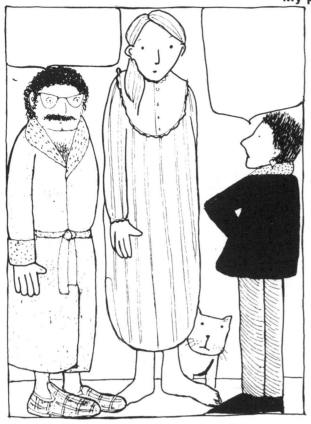 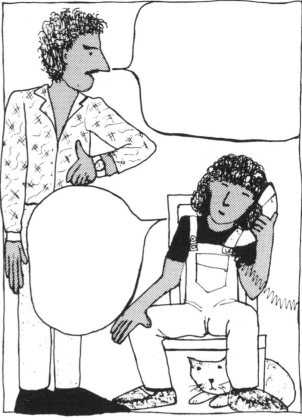

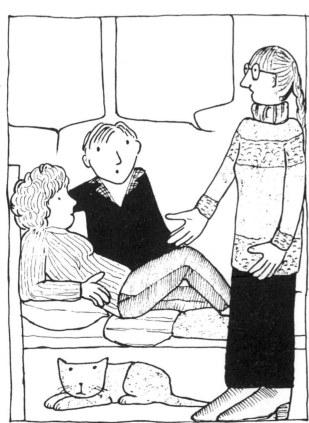 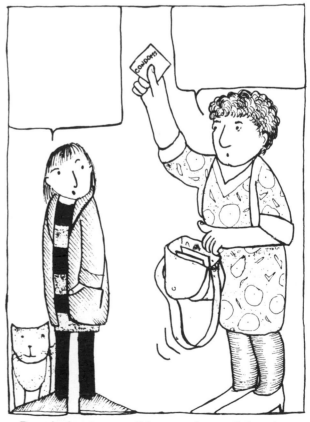

# 36 The family - values voting

| | |
|---|---|
| **Objectives** | To make a public statement about the family.<br>To move and have fun. |
| **Prerequisites** | None. |
| **Age group** | 13-16, 16 + |
| **Group size** | Ideally a maximum of 25. |
| **Time needed** | 15 minutes. |
| **What you need** | Nothing. |

**How you do it**

a  Explain that you will read out a statement and that people should respond quickly with hand signals, without too much thought or debate. It is an instant reaction and represents how a person thinks right now. Later their answers may well be different.

b  Explain the hand signals (page 35).

c  Read the statements. In this activity it is useful for the educator to participate, but delay your voting slightly, because it is possible for you to influence group members.

▶ **Suggested statements about families**
A family is a group of people living together.
A family consists of a mother, father and children.
A family is parents, grandparents, relatives and children.
Families should have at least one meal together each day.
Adults have the right to decide how their children should behave.
Sex education should only come from parents.
Teenagers should be able to decide whom they go out with.

| | |
|---|---|
| **Variation** | This activity can be used in almost every area of human relationships. Design a range of statements to suit your needs. However, always start with non-threatening statements and move towards the more difficult. |
| **Note** | This is a good opening activity and it is not necessary to have follow-up discussion unless it seems appropriate. |

# 37 The family — values ranking

| | |
|---|---|
| **Objective** | To clarify values and attitudes about families. |
| **Prerequisites** | None. |
| **Age group** | 13-16, 16 + |
| **Group size** | Ideally a maximum of 25. |
| **Time needed** | 15-20 minutes. |
| **What you need** | Prepared statement (see examples below). |

**How you do it**

a Explain that you will be reading out a statement with 3 choices. These must be ranked in order from most important (1) to least important (3).

b Read out the statements and the choices slowly. Repeat them.

c Ask those participants who are willing, to share their rankings with the group. It is important to observe the right to pass.

d Continue until all statements are finished.

e Discuss the general attitudes expressed about the family and the values that are implied by these attitudes.

▶**Suggested statements**

a The most important thing about a family is that it provides:
love and care
security and protection
friendship and understanding

b Brothers and sisters should always:
stick together
share things
mind their own business

**Variation**  The statement and choices can be pre-written with a copy for the participants to complete their own private rankings.

# 38 Jenny's dilemma

| | |
|---|---|
| **Objectives** | To commence learning the skills of decision-making and problem-solving. To learn how to identify the problem in a situation and to be able to translate the above skills into day to day living. |
| **Prerequisites** | None. |
| **Age group** | 13-16, 16 + <br> This activity could be adapted for 9-13 year olds. |
| **Group size** | Ideally a maximum of 25. |
| **Time needed** | 45 minutes. |
| **What you need** | A copy of the story for each participant (page 85) and large sheets of paper hung around the room. |

**How you do it**

a  Hand out a copy of the story to each participant and read it aloud. Pose the question:
'What should Jenny do?'

b  Ask the participants to brainstorm (page 21) a list of possible actions Jenny can take. Write each suggestion on the top of a new sheet of paper.

c  When the ideas are exhausted, draw a line down the centre of each page, so that the possible outcomes of each action can be written in positive or negative columns.

d  Working on one action at a time, ask the participants to suggest possible outcomes and write these in the appropriate column. Treat all suggestions seriously.

e  When all the lists are finished, take each action and its possible outcomes, and through discussion start to eliminate those actions which seem unrealistic or unreasonable.

f  Identify the three most likely courses of action and then discuss these in small groups. Try to reach a consensus about the best possible solution.

**Note**  This process can be used to solve dilemmas that arise in the group and for individuals who raise a problem for discussion.

# Jenny's dilemma

Jenny is 21, Sue is 15, and they are sisters. They have often had problems with each other. Jenny resents the relative freedom that their parents allow Sue. When she was 15, Jenny's parents kept a close eye on where she went and who she went with, but now they seem much more easygoing with Sue. Sue resents the fact that Jenny has more privileges than her, and that she has an income and all the freedom she likes. Also, Sue is still dependent on her parents for money, and they do not let her come and go as she pleases.

Jenny is attending courses at night school. One evening she is on her way home, when she hears a smash, and the street light goes out. As she draws closer to the group on the street she sees Sue is one of the group and that they are throwing stones at the street light. Jenny is furious and goes to Sue and says, 'I'm going home to tell Mum and Dad right now what their little darling does with her wonderful friends'.

Sue is really upset. She says to Jenny, 'If you tell Mum and Dad, I'll leave home right now. I know what I'm doing and I don't want you interfering in my life'.

What should Jenny do?

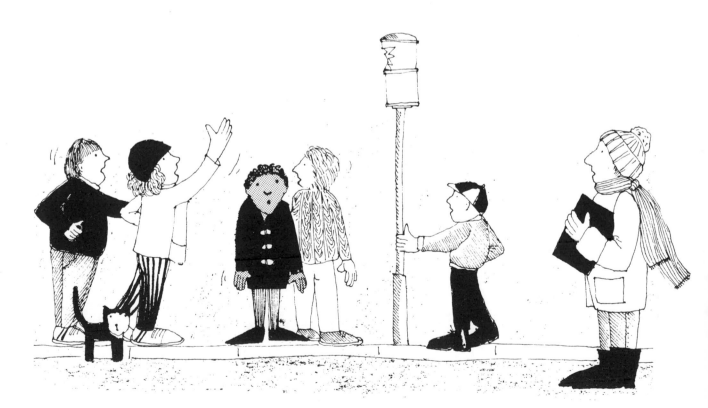

# 39 Dear heart

| | |
|---|---|
| **Objectives** | To provide an opportunity for discussion on relationship problems.<br>To develop problem-solving strategies. |
| **Prerequisites** | Positive support in the group. |
| **Age group** | 13-16, 16 + |
| **Group size** | Ideally a maximum of 25. |
| **Time needed** | 30 minutes. |
| **What you need** | Paper, pens, letters cut from advice columns in popular magazines with replies omitted.<br>Select letters that are appropriate to the group. |

**How you do it**

a  Divide the group into groups of 3 or 4.

b  Hand out a letter to each group and ask them to play the part of the adviser.
Allow 10-15 minutes to write an answer to the letter.

c  Re-form the large group and ask the small groups to share their problem letters and replies.

d  Focus discussion on the replies.
Were they practical?
Were they sympathetic?
Were there any other solutions?

**Variation**  Ask individuals in the group to write their own 'problem' letters and deposit them into a central mailbag. Groups or individuals then draw out a letter and reply as above.

**Note**  The group needs to be sensitive and caring for this variation, as a real problem handled carelessly could be compounded for the writer.

# **40** The problem page

|  |  |
|---|---|
| | For use with 'Boy and Girl' from the film series 'Loving and Caring'. |
| **Objectives** | To explore in a group some of the dilemmas experienced by young people faced with the decision of whether or not to have sexual intercourse.<br>To stimulate discussion about sexual decision making. |
| **Prerequisites** | A feeling of trust and acceptance. |
| **Age group** | 13-16, 16 + |
| **Group size** | Ideally a maximum of 25. |
| **Time needed** | 45 minutes which includes time for viewing the film. |
| **What you need** | Writing materials, a projector or video and screen, the film 'Loving and Caring part one: Boy and Girl'. |

**How you do it**

a Show the film.

b Divide into small groups after the film. Before any discussion, explain that each group is going to be the author of a magazine advice column.

c The groups are to consider the situation portrayed in the film and imagine that they have a letter asking for advice from either Sandra or Simon. Their task is to write a reply advising Sandra or Simon on what they should do. Designate groups to reply to either Sandra or Simon.

d Allow 15-20 minutes for each group to write a reply.

e When the replies are written, re-form the total group and ask each of the groups to read their advice.

f When all replies have been read, focus discussion on the responses.
Is there agreement in the group?
What are the sources of disagreement?
What are the dilemmas faced by Sandra?
What are the dilemmas faced by Simon?
Do these situations happen in real life?
How can similar situations be handled?

**Variation**

After step d, pass the replies around so that each group presents another group's response. This provides opportunity to explore diversity of opinions.

**Note**

This film is also available on video (see page 196).

# **41** Women, men and society

| | |
|---|---|
| **Objectives** | To identify sex role stereotypes. |
| | To provide the opportunity for discussion on alternatives to traditional sex roles. |
| | To explore attitudes towards female and male roles. |
| | To discuss the effects of sex roles on relationships. |
| **Prerequisites** | Literacy skills. |
| **Age group** | 13-16, 16 + |
| **Group size** | Ideally a maximum of 25. |
| **Time needed** | 45 minutes. |
| **What you need** | Large sheets of paper, felt-tip pens, space for four groups to work separately. |

**How you do it**

a  Divide the large group into four groups, each with paper and pens.

b  Ask each group to appoint a recorder and someone to report back to the whole group.

c  Instruct the first group to list all the advantages of being a woman in our society;
the second group to list all the advantages of being a man;
the third group to list all the disadvantages of being a woman;
and the fourth group to list all the disadvantages of being a man.

d  After 15-20 minutes, or when the groups have all finished, re-form the large group. The small groups are then asked to display and read their lists to the large group.

e  Note the similarities and differences between the lists.

f  Discuss the following questions:
Are people limited by roles, and why?
Are the roles interchangeable?
What are the benefits of sex roles, and who benefits?
How do sex roles affect relationships?
What would group members like to change?

# 42 Media images: collage

| | |
|---|---|
| **Objectives** | To examine images of women and men as portrayed in the media. To stimulate discussion on these images and how they maintain sex role stereotypes. |
| **Prerequisites** | None. |
| **Age group** | 13-16, 16 + |
| **Group size** | Ideally a maximum of 25. |
| **Time needed** | 50 minutes to 1 hour. |
| **What you need** | A variety of magazines and newspapers, glue, large sheets of paper, sticky tape, scissors. |

**How you do it**

a  Divide into small groups of 3 or 4 participants.

b  Provide each group with the necessary materials to create a collage.

c  Ask half of the small groups to prepare collages of the way women are portrayed in the media. Ask the other groups to prepare collages of the way men are portrayed.

d  After about 30 minutes or when the collages are completed, bring the groups together so that they may share their work and describe the images they found.

e  Discussion may include: the different images, how these images maintain sex role stereotypes, and how they affect human behaviour and relationships. Also discuss the accuracy of the images and how participants feel about being portrayed in this way.

**Follow-up**

Assign the participants to watch two films and ask them to observe sex role stereotypes. Discuss their experiences in a later session.

**Variation**

Collages may be made by collecting images of girls and boys instead of women and men.

# **43** Re-sexing the ads

| | |
|---|---|
| **Objectives** | To critically examine the way the media, through advertising confirms and reinforces sex role stereotypes. |
| | To provide an opportunity for small groups to express themselves creatively through drama. |
| **Prerequisites** | Mixed group. Awareness of current T.V. advertisements. |
| **Age group** | 9-13, 13-16, 16+ |
| **Group size** | Ideally a maximum of 25. |
| **Time needed** | 45 minutes to 1 hour. |
| **What you need** | Nothing. |
| **How you do it** | |

a  Ask the group to think about television advertisements in which both women and men are portrayed.

b  Divide into small groups.

c  Ask the groups to develop sketches and act out the advertisements of their choice, with gender reversed. Males play female parts, females play male parts. The sketch is to remain faithful to the content and spirit of the advertisement.

d  After the groups have had enough time to prepare, they take turns to perform for the rest of the group.

e  When all the sketches have been performed, re-form the group and focus discussion on the observations and feelings in the group:
How did it feel as a male to play a female role?
How did it feel as a female to play a male role?
Was it funny?
Why?
What is sex role stereotyping?
Why does it exist?
Is it important?
What can be done to counter it?

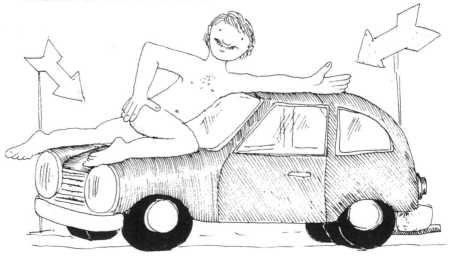

# **44** Discussion sheets

| | |
|---|---|
| **Objectives** | To trigger discussion on specific, complex social issues related to sexuality.<br>To generate a range of questions and comments about these issues and to provide opportunities to further explore them. |
| **Prerequisites** | Literacy skills. |
| **Age group** | 16 + |
| **Group size** | Ideally a maximum of 25. |
| **Time needed** | 40-50 minutes. |
| **What you need** | A copy of the relevant discussion sheet (pages 92-94) for each participant. |

**How you do it**

a Hand out copies of the discussion sheet.

b Ask the participants to read the statements on their sheets and prepare lists of questions or comments that they wish to make about the topic.

c Divide the large group into small groups for discussion. Have each small group appoint a recorder and proceed to make a composite list of questions, comments and reactions.

d When the lists are complete, have the recorder report the major points to the total group.

e Answer any questions and focus discussion on attitudes expressed, myths and misconceptions, and areas of concern.

| | |
|---|---|
| **Follow-up** | Explore any questions that are difficult to answer, and further research the subject by visits and community contacts to relevant agencies, guest speakers, panel discussions, films, videos, projects and readings. |
| **Variation** | After step c, continue discussion using debating rules or a fishbowl format (page 20). |

# Discussion sheets

### Sexuality and ageing

There are lot of ways in which our society simply ignores elderly people. Yet surely a couple who have experienced joys, sorrows and intimacy together for maybe 30 or 40 years have something special to share with young people just starting out on relationships?

'Ageism is the idea that people become inferior, different and somehow dehumanised by virtue of having lived a specified number of years. Ageism is a prejudice like racism, which is based on fear, folklore and the hang-ups of a few people who propagate these prejudices. Like racism, it needs to be countered by information, contradiction and confrontation. The people who are the target of the prejudice have to stand up for themselves in order to put it down.'

Old people deserve privacy and the opportunity to establish relationships when and with whom they wish. Why do people find shocking the idea of a 70 year-old who still wants an active sex life? Doesn't s/he have the same rights as any other responsible adult?

### Masturbation

'Masturbation is a common sexual activity that is usually enjoyable. The vast majority of people do it regardless of other sexual activity.'

'Many people still believe that masturbation is wrong. In the past, people believed that masturbation could cause blindness, insanity, sterility, or hairs to grow on their palms. Many church teachings still say that masturbation is a sin.'

'Many people, especially younger people, think they are the only ones who masturbate or that they masturbate too much. This can be a worrying idea.'

'For many people, masturbation is a positive way of finding out about their bodies, and what gives them pleasure.'

'Girls and women can enjoy masturbating; it is not only boys and men who masturbate.'

It's okay not to masturbate too. There's nothing wrong if you don't.

# Discussion sheets

## Lesbianism

'Many lesbians have had sexual relationships with men, and some have been, and still are, married. Being a lesbian does not necessarily mean hating men — many lesbians still have close friendships with men.'

'There are no specific laws against lesbianism because the people who made the laws didn't believe that it existed. Women have been loving and caring for each other for centuries. Sometimes this is sexual, sometimes not.'

'People sometimes ask what makes a women a lesbian. It's as easy to ask what makes a women a heterosexual.'

'Life is not always easy for lesbians. Often they have to hide their feelings and lie about their close relationships and social life. There are many situations in which it would be impossible to admit to being a lesbian, so they need to think about everything they say.'

'Being a lesbian means loving other women.'

'For some women, being a lesbian isn't just a personal thing, it's also a political statement. Many lesbians believe that they are stronger as women by not relating sexually with men. They feel that they can be more independent individuals.'

## Male homosexuality

'Kissing is accepted between heterosexual people. It is an expression of affection between homosexual people as well. If you accept gay people, you accept their behaviour too.'

'Is it moral or immoral? I don't know. Can I judge? I do know that my son's homosexual relationship is a loving, caring, faithful one. What more could I want?'

'Men may express their homosexuality in a number of different ways, at different times and in varying degrees. As for the causes of homosexuality — why is there a need to find a cause? No-one ever asks what causes heterosexuality,'

More people now believe that homosexuals, lesbians and heterosexuals should have the same rights, yet a person who openly acknowledges being gay still runs the risk of alienating family, friends and colleagues. Why is it that some people find lesbians and homosexuals threatening? Why can't the law treat them like everyone else — as individuals who fall in love and have relationships, and want to live their lives free from discrimination and guilt?

# Discussion sheets

## Bisexuality

'David Bowie, Bette Midler and Boy George all display a prominent stage image of bisexuality. They aim to be attractive to both women and men. Successful musicals such as Hair and the Rocky Horror Show mock conventional sexuality and show the possibilities of bisexuality.

'Bisexuality is the ability to love, and to express that love with both women and men. Most people are socialised into a role which carries with it loving people of the opposite sex. Many reject this role, or never accept it, and love people of the same sex. A few fit into both groups.'

'Why can't people love others as people first, responding to sexuality as a part of being human?'

## Celibacy

'Celibacy in the past has been viewed as a temporary and transient state, except for those who choose it as a religious discipline. Celibacy is not an alternative that many people elect voluntarily. For those who do, it must be viewed as an honourable and viable alternative for life, or for any period a person decides upon. It also does not exclude physical closeness or intimacy with other people, or a long term domestic relationship. Celibacy can be practised in and outside of marriage.'

'I enjoy the company of the opposite sex; I am attracted to them and they to me. Since I am not interested at the moment in a sex-based relationship I try not to make myself available.'

'Many sexual relationships are based on one partner exerting power over the other and on domination and oppression. To honestly try to change, these kinds of relationships may require an agreement for each person to remain celibate for an extended period, until they are able to relate to each other as equals.'

'Some people come to identify that they don't need sexual intercourse. For these people celibacy is desirable, even preferable to intercourse.'

# Exploitation in relationships

We are very conscious that some of the most difficult topics in sex education are those which involve exploitation. We have quite deliberately not included rape, pornography, incest and prostitution in any other part of this manual, because we see them as exploitation, violence and denial of sexuality. We have also found it extremely difficult to develop strategies which adequately deal with these topics.

Nevertheless, we believe that it is vital for educators to explore these issues with young people. Within any group there may be victims of exploitation. Your sessions may be the only opportunity for young people to discuss these sensitive topics in a supportive environment. Open discussion provides an opportunity to dispel misconceptions and replace them with information.

It is vital for more work to be done by educators so that they can enhance their own understanding of these difficult issues as well as develop activities that are effective in assisting young people.

We have had some success in using Discussion Sheets (pages 91-97) as an introduction to these topics.

## References

Brown Miller, S., *Against Our Will: Men, Women, and Rape*, Bantam, 1975
CIBA Foundation, *Child Sexual Abuse within the Family*, Tavistock Publications, 1984
Elliott, M., *Preventing Child Sexual Assault: A Practical Guide to Talking with Children*, Bedford Square Press/NCVO, 1985
Forward, S. and Buck, C., *Betrayal of Innocence: Incest and its Devastation*, Penguin, 1981
Griffin, S., *Pornography and Silence*, The Women's Press, 1981
London Rape Crisis Centre, *Sexual Violence: The Reality for Women*, The Women's Press, 1984
Millett, K., *The Prostitution Papers*, Paladin, 1975

## Videos/Films
Feeling Yes, Feeling No
Kids Can Say No!
Say No To Strangers

# Exploitation in relationships

## Incest

'Historically, the taboo against incest was a way of ensuring children left the family and made links with others, thus providing the security of family networks.'

'Incest is a very emotional subject. For the victims there can be feelings of shame, humiliation, guilt, anger and confusion — for others in the family, feelings of hostility and misunderstanding.'

Incest is when a parent, relative, brother or anyone in the family in a position of power and trust sexually abuses one or more members of that same family. Sexual abuse is not love and it is not affection. It is a denial of the rights of the abused.

'Incest is not talked about. People don't want to be involved. It's hard to get someone to listen. So who can a victim turn to?'

'The most common form of incest, that between father and daughter, is now recognised as a form of child abuse.'

'To some people, incest is a grave and dreaded sin that is too horrifying to talk about.'

## Rape

'Rape is not about sex. If sex is about caring for another person and about mutual pleasure, then violently attacking another person, enjoying humiliating and terrifying them or beating them up is just the opposite of sex. Rape is about power and violence.'

'All men benefit from the violent oppression of women by a few men.'

'Women have learnt to see themselves as weak and men as strong. As a result of this, women do not feel they have the power to do anything about rape.'

'Not all men rape women. But what happens if you are on your way home at night, and you see a man or a group of men walking towards you? What do you do? Cross the road? Walk faster and look straight ahead? Ignore them, but feel scared all the same? It doesn't really matter if they are decent men because in that kind of situation you can't tell. Every man you meet *is* someone to be scared of because he is a man. As long as some men attack women, then every woman has to be frightened of, or at least wary of every man.'

'Many women who are raped by their husbands do not see themselves as victims of rape.'

'Each time a woman is raped, society and every individual in it is responsible. We are at the same time victim and attacker. If we know about the problems and don't respond by trying to change a society that makes it possible, we are just as responsible as the rapist.'

'Most of us believe that rapists are violent strangers. This is not always true. The vast majority of women are raped in their own homes by men they know.'

# Exploitation in relationships

## Pornography

'Viewing pornography can influence us in our behaviour towards each other.'

'Pornography distorts reality by showing women and men as physically stereotyped and unreal. It portrays relationships and situations that would be unacceptable and emotionally unsatisfying to most people.'

'In the past, pornography was defined as the display of naked bodies, and of people having sex. This made objects of women. A different kind of pornography is emerging now, which not only degrades women, but also involves violence and humiliation.'

'Pornography makes money for a few people at the expense of many.'

## Prostitution

'Many women who become prostitutes do so to earn an income. If they could earn a similar amount in another way, they would probably give up prostitution.'

'Men have sex with prostitutes to prove their masculinity, sexual ability, or to demonstrate their power over women.'

'Our society is two-faced in its attitude to prostitution. The woman in a doorway or under a lamppost is regarded as offensive and socially unacceptable. It is not seen as offensive for men to hoot from a car, whistle from a building site, leer from the kerbside or jostle women on the street, and offer those women a price.'

'The law is harsher on prostitutes than their customers. In some places it is against the law for a prostitute to solicit, or accept a customer, but it is not against the law for the customer to ask for services.'

Permission to copy this page for participant use.

# Sexual decision making

## Factors to Consider
Social influences, emotional influences, legal issues, decision-making, options and consequences, unplanned pregnancy.

## Words the Educator May Want to Know and Understand
Assertiveness, communication, responsibility, choices, guilt, exploitation, sexual feelings, love, peer pressure, parental attitudes and influences, parenting, rights of mother, rights of father, unplanned pregnancy, wanted pregnancy, unwanted pregnancy, childless by choice, single parenthood, marriage, age of consent, carnal knowledge.

## References
Bury, J., *Teenage Pregnancy in Britain*, Birth Control Trust, 1984
Dickson, A., *A Woman in Your Own Right*, Quartet, 1982

## Reading for Participants
Dickson, A., *A Woman in Your Own Right*, Quartet, 1982
Rayner, C., *Growing Pains — and How To Avoid Them*, Corgi, 1984

## Videos/Films
Danny's Big Night
If Only We'd Known
Loving and Caring
One in 44
Sex and Sensibility
Somebody's Daughter
Sweet Sixteen and Pregnant
Teenage Father

## Additional Resources
Abortion
Discussion Cards
The Grapevine Game
It's Your Life: Babies and Parents
Lifeskills Teaching Programme No. 3
Living Choices
Male and Female (CRAC)
Why Discuss Abortion?

## Activities
45  Decisions, decisions . . .
46  What are the options?
47  How to say no
48  Re-write the story
49  Can you handle it?
50  If I had a baby
51  What would others think?
52  Sexual messages

# 45 Decisions, decisions

| | |
|---|---|
| **Objectives** | To enable the participants to make a public statement about issues relating to relationships.<br>To work on clarifying the attitudes expressed in the public statement. |
| **Prerequisites** | Positive support within the group. |
| **Age group** | 13-16, 16 + |
| **Group size** | Ideally a maximum of 25. |
| **Time needed** | 20-30 minutes. |
| **What you need** | Three large cards marked *A, B* and *C*.<br>3 or 4 prepared statements (see suggestions below). |

**How you do it**

a Place the cards *A, B* and *C* in three corners of the room.

b Explain that you are going to read out some statements about relationships. Each of the statements has three options, and participants are to choose one option and move to the corner which represents the response with which they most agree. Stress that participants may choose to pass, and to indicate this they stand in the centre of the room with their arms folded.

c Read the statements twice, instructing the participants to move without discussion to the corner that best describes their current response.

d Now read one of the statements.
If I ate out I would prefer:
to have a hamburger with a group of friends and pay for myself.—Go to *A*.
to go to the best restaurant in town and be paid for.—Go to *B*.
to go to my friend's house and eat with the family.—Go to *C*.

e In order to briefly discuss their options, have the participants
turn to another person in the same corner or
form sub-groups of 3 or 4 or
find a partner from another corner or
allow volunteers from each corner to make a personal statement to the entire group.

▶ **Suggested statements**
1 I would prefer to:
spend an evening with a close friend .................................................... *A*
spend a day outdoors alone .................................................... *B*
go out with the person of my dreams .................................................... *C*
2 If I were sexually active I would most want my relationship to be:
enjoyable .................................................... *A*
open and honest .................................................... *B*
mutually satisfying .................................................... *C*
3 The worst thing I could find out about my partner (girlfriend or boyfriend, wife or husband), would be that:
she or he were sterile .................................................... *A*
she or he were promiscuous .................................................... *B*
she or he had a sexually transmitted disease .................................................... *C*

**Note** The educator needs to choose statements that are relevant to the group.

# 46 What are the options?

| | |
|---|---|
| **Objective** | To encourage participants to look at a range of options for sexual behaviour including those with which she or he may not agree. |
| **Prerequisites** | None |
| **Age group** | 13-16, 16 + |
| **Group size** | Minimum of 10, maximum of 25. |
| **Time needed** | 45 minutes to 1 hour. |
| **What you need** | Large sheets of paper, felt-tip pens. |

**How you do it**

a  Divide the large group into 5 small groups of equal size.

b  Allocate one of the following options to each group:
not being sexually active
just kissing, and holding hands
sexual activity without penetrative sex
having sexual intercourse without using a condom
having sexual intercourse using a condom

c  Ask the groups to list all the advantages and disadvantages of their specific option for self and (if relevant) for partner.

d  Each small group reports back to the large group.

**Follow-up**

1  Give each person a list of the options and ask them to develop a private list of advantages and disadvantages for them personally.

2  An additional activity would be to explore the options available for unplanned pregnancy — abortion, adoption or fostering, single parent-hood, marriage.

3  Set each group to research factual information on options such as:
availability of contraception
incidence of unplanned pregnancy, abortion, adoption etc.
support structures
cost of each option

Report findings to the large group in the next session.

**Note**     It may be necessary as a preliminary to this activity, to discuss the meaning of the options.

# 47 How to say no

| | |
|---|---|
| **Objectives** | To expose the lines often used by young men to pressure young women into sexual activity.<br>To give female participants the opportunity to practise assertive responses to these every day (night) lines. |
| **Prerequisites** | None. |
| **Age group** | 13-16, 16 + |
| **Group size** | Ideally a maximum of 25. |
| **Time needed** | 45 minutes. |
| **What you need** | Large sheets of paper, felt-tip pens, sticky tape, display area. |
| **How you do it** | |

a Divide the group into small, single-sex groups of 3 or 4.

b Using the rules for brainstorming (page 21) generate a list of all the common lines that participants have ever heard.

c Ask each group to read out its list and then display them around the room.

d Divide the group into pairs but not necessarily female and male. One of the partners selects a line from the list and the other devises an impromptu response.

e Allow 10-15 minutes for the pairs to take turns practising their responses to the lines and keeping a note of them.

f Ask each pair to select any particularly interesting response to share with the large group.

g Discussion in the large group may focus on the following points:
coping with rejection
decision-making on sexual matters
sex roles
how to communicate sexual needs and wants as equals

▶ **Suggested lines**

Everyone else does it.

You're the only person I've ever done this with.

You won't get pregnant if we do it standing up.

You might as well do it — I'll tell everyone you did anyway.

This is the way to prove you really love me.

You got me all excited, now it's up to you to do something about it.

**Variations**

1 Similar lines can be devised for other topics such as birth control and sexually transmitted diseases.

2 For larger numbers, this activity can be done in small groups instead of pairs, with one person reading the line and the rest of the group taking turns to respond.

# 48 Re-write the story

| | |
|---|---|
| **Objectives** | To encourage creative problem-solving and decision-making in the area of sexuality.<br>To foster the acceptance of a range of solutions to a specific problem.<br>To discuss personal and social issues relating to sexual intercourse. |
| **Prerequisites** | None. |
| **Age group** | 16 + |
| **Time needed** | 40-60 minutes. |
| **What you need** | A copy of the story *Bob and Carol, Ted and Alice, and Mrs Davis* (page 103) for each small group. A small card for each participant, labelled with a character's name from the story. |

**How you do it**

a  Ask the participants to form groups of six to match the number of characters in the story.

b  Give each group a copy of the story and give each person a card indicating which character she or he is to role-play. The sex of the participant does not have to match that of the character.

c  Tell them they are to re-write the story — work out what they would like to have happen, and then prepare a role-play (pages 23-24).

d  Allow 15 minutes to prepare the story.

e  Each group will then present its role-play to the other groups. Allow 10 minutes for each group.

f  Derole and debrief (page 24).

g  Discuss the issues which have arisen from the role-plays. Some which may emerge are:
age of sexual encounters
types of sexual encounters
attitudes of doctors to young people requesting contraception
love
parental attitudes and influences
alcohol
unwanted pregnancy
women's roles
what is socially acceptable
risk of HIV infection/AIDS

| | |
|---|---|
| **Follow-up** | Use *What are the options?* (page 100) to discuss Carol's situation. |
| **Variation** | Instead of re-writing the story, ask the groups to write and role-play an ending to the existing story. |

# Bob and Carol, Ted and Alice, and Mrs Davis

**Characters: Alice, family doctor, Bob, Carol, Mrs Davis, Ted**

Alice is just about half-way between her sixteenth and seventeenth birthdays. She is very attractive and also popular with the boys in her school. For some time she has been worrying that she might get pregnant. So one day she visited her family doctor and explained to him that she wanted to go on the pill. He asked her if she were going steady with anyone and Alice said yes she was, and she knew that she needed to be responsible. The doctor gave her a prescription for the pill and Alice began taking it as instructed.

One of the fellows Alice went out with pretty often was Bob. She liked him a lot, and he thought she was really smashing looking. But what he liked best was that he didn't have to talk her into sex every time they went out — since she was on the pill, Alice was willing, and they always ended up having intercourse. Though Alice went out with other boys, she liked Bob the best, and was in love with him. Bob liked Alice, liked her availability even more, but was not in love with her at all. He would sleep with her as often as he could.

When Alice went on the pill, she naturally told her best friend, Carol. Carol told her mother, Mrs Davis, that Alice was on the pill and her mother was both angry and upset. She told Carol that the friendship with Alice must be broken off immediately and that Carol was not to have anything further to do with Alice. Though Mrs Davis took the line with Carol that any girl who was on the pill was one to stay away from, her real fear was that Alice would influence Carol into going on the pill. Carol gave in to her mother's wishes and broke off her long time friendship with Alice.

Carol had been going steady with Ted for almost two years. They had indulged in some sexual play but Carol was insistent that she did not want to go 'all the way'. Ted really wanted to have intercourse with Carol, so one night at a party he got her very drunk, suspecting that she would be willing. Carol was too drunk to know what she was doing and that night Carol and Ted had sexual intercourse. As a result of that one experience Carol is pregnant. She has told Ted, but no one else. Ted is willing to marry her. Carol is seventeen; Ted is eighteen.

Mrs Davis, Carol's mother, is very ambitious for Carol. At any rate she wants Carol to have more out of life than she had. What she fears more than anything else is that Carol will waste herself on someone socially unacceptable, such as Ted.

# 49 Can you handle it?

**Objective**
To provide an opportunity for the participants to learn about some of the responsibilities associated with having a baby.

**Prerequisites**
None.

**Age group**
13-16, 16 +

**Group size**
Ideally a maximum of 25.

**Time needed**
20 minutes to explain the activity.
1 week to carry out the activity.
30 minutes for follow-up discussion.

**What you need**
1 raw egg for each person, paper, pens.

**How you do it**

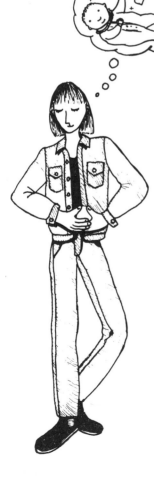

a  Explain that this activity is practice in caring for an imaginary baby. The egg will represent the baby.

b  Give the following instructions and rules for the care of the egg (baby):

Assume total responsibility for the egg.

Keep it warm and give it fresh air daily.

If the egg has to be left, it must be in the care of another responsible person and payment arranged, either monetary or a reciprocal agreement.

Should any disaster befall the egg, a pre-arranged fine must be paid to an agreed cause, and a period of mourning observed for two days. At the end of this period, replace the egg.

A daily diary must be kept on all activities, the care given, and how the participant felt about the egg and the experiment.

c  Explain that the experiment will continue for a full week, and that participants are expected to act responsibly and take the activity seriously. (Not everyone will, but it can be interesting to discuss the reasons why at the end.)

d  Set the time and place for reporting back to discuss and evaluate the activity.

# 50 If I had a baby

**Objectives**     To provide an opportunity for participants to identify the changes they would need to make in their activities if they had a baby.
To promote discussion on the responsibilities associated with parenting.

**Prerequisites**     Literacy skills.

**Age group**     13-16, 16 +

**Group size**     Ideally a maximum of 25.

**Time needed**     30-45 minutes.

**What you need**     Paper, pens.

**How you do it**

a  Hand out paper and pens to each participant.

b  Ask participants to divide their pages in half lengthways.

c  In the left half of the page have them list twelve things that they really like to do. They may have more or less than twelve, the number is not important. Stress that the lists are personal as they will not have to share them.

d  When the lists are completed ask participants to make four columns on the right side of the page.

e  Then ask them to code their lists as instructed below. Give one instruction at a time, allowing time between each for completion of coding.

f  Ask the participants to write a pound sign in the first column opposite anything on their lists that costs more than three pounds.
In the second column, write *A* for anything that is done alone or *P* for anything that is done with other people.
In the third column write *D* for day, *W* for week, *M* for month, *Y* for year, for the length of time since the activity was undertaken.
In the last column write *B* for anything that would be difficult to do with a three month old baby.

g  When the coding is completed, ask the participants to review their lists and think about some of the following questions:
Are there any patterns?
Is there anything you would like to change?
How many activities would you still be able to do with a young baby?
Were there any surprises?

h  Have each participant complete the following sentences stems:
I was surprised to find that . . .
I became aware that . . .

i  In small groups share and discuss the completed sentences.

# 51 What would others think?

**Objectives**   To allow participants to consider the reactions of the significant people in their lives regarding the issue of unplanned pregnancy.
To help participants explore their own feelings about being pregnant or having a partner who is pregnant.

**Prerequisites**   Positive support in the group.

**Age group**   13-16, 16+

**Group size**   Ideally a maximum of 25.

**Time needed**   20-30 minutes.

**What you need**   Paper and pen for each participant.

**How you do it**

a   Explain that this is a private activity and sharing will only occur if individuals choose.

b   Ask participants to divide their pages into five equal columns, as shown below. Then write the name of her or his:
best friend at the top of the first column;
parent or guardian at the top of the second column;
own name at the top of the third column;
favourite adult at the top of the fourth column;
partner (girlfriend or boyfriend) at the top of the fifth column.

| Amy | Dad | Me (Helen) | Nana | Jo |
|---|---|---|---|---|
|  |  |  |  |  |

c   In the centre column marked 'Me', ask participants to write how they might feel and react to being pregnant or having a partner who is pregnant.

d   Write in each of the other columns how the others might feel and react to this pregnancy.

e   On the back of the page, ask participants to complete a sentence stem such as:
I found that I . . .
I felt that I . . .
I was surprised to find that I . . .

f   Form into small groups and share the results of the sentence stems.

g   In the large group, discuss the general reactions to unplanned pregnancy.

# 52 Sexual messages

**Objectives**
To identify the sexual 'messages' participants have received.
To explore ways in which these have affected participants' attitudes, behaviour and values.
To look at the choices participants can make about their future.

**Prerequisites**
A feeling of trust and acceptance.

**Age group**
16 +

**Group size**
Any size.

**Time needed**
1 hour.

**What you need**
Paper and pen for each participant, space for private work, a quiet environment.

**How to do it**

a  Choose a partner with whom you feel happy to share some personal thoughts and feelings. Stress that the first part of this activity is private.

b  Ask each participant to represent on their paper the 'messages' they have received (or things they have learnt) to do with relationships and sex. These may be about information, sexual identity, sexual behaviour, responsibilities, expectations etc. The representation may be in words, pictures, diagrams or symbols.

It may help to remind them that messages may have been verbal or non-verbal (what was not said may be as important as what was said); the messages may have come from parents, siblings, peers, the media; and they begin at birth and go on being received.

Allow about 15 minutes for this.

c  Ask participants to share what they choose of this in pairs.

d  Ask participants to divide the 'messages' they received about sex into three groups:
— those that no longer affect their lives.
— those that are still significant, and affect their lives negatively.
— those that are still significant, and affect their lives positively.

e  Ask participants to share in pairs how their lives are affected by these messages and what changes they would like to make.

**Follow-up**

1  Ask participants to complete the following sentences:

I learned that I . . .
I was surprised to find that I . . .
I hope that I . . .

and share them in small groups.

2  Write a change contract on the lines of *Promises to myself* (page 74).

107

# My body myself

## Factors to Consider
Anatomy and physiology of the female and male reproductive systems, body image, sensuality, sexuality, sexual maturity, sexual response, appropriateness of social norms, sexual responsibility, terminology — medical and common.

## Words the Educator May Want to Know and Understand
### Female Reproductive System
Ampulla, Bartholin's glands, breasts, cervix, cilia, clitoris, Fallopian tubes, fimbria, genitalia, gonad, hormones, hymen, labia majora, labia minora, ligaments, menstrual cycle, mons pubis, os, ovaries, pelvis, perineum, pubic hair, urethra, uterus, vagina, vestibule, vulva.

### Male Reproductive System
Bladder, Bulbo-urethral glands (Cowper's glands), circumcision, cremasteric muscle, descent of testes, ejaculation, ejaculatory duct, epididymis, erection, foreskin, frenulum, glans, gonad, inguinal canal, penis, prepuce, prostate gland, scrotum, semen, seminal vesicles, seminiferous tubules, smegma, sperm, spermatogenesis, spermatozoa, testes, urethra, vas deferens.

### Glands and Hormones
Androgen, anterior pituitary gland, follicle stimulating hormones (FSH), gonadatrophins, hypothalamus, interstitial cell stimulating hormone, luteinising hormone (LH), oestrogen, progesterone, releasing factors, testosterone.

### Sexual Response
Arousal, brain, central nervous system, climax, consummation, cunnilingus, enjoyment, erogenous zones, excitement, fellatio, foreplay, frigidity, hearing, impotence, libido, masturbation, orgasm, plateau, refactory phase, resolution, sexual intercourse, sight, smell, taste, virgin.

## References
Belliveau, F. and Richter, L., *Understanding Human Sexual Inadequacy*, Hodder (Paperbacks), 1971
Hite, S., *The Hite Report on Female Sexuality*, Corgi, 1981
Kitzinger, S., *Woman's Experiences of Sex*, Penguin, 1985
Phillips, A. and Rakusen, J., *Our Bodies Ourselves*, Penguin, 1989
Zilbergeld, B., *Men and Sex*, Fontana, 1986

### Readings for Participants

Claesson, B. H., *Boy, Girl, Man, Woman: A Guide to Sex for Young People*, Penguin, 1979
(This book was written for young people, but some educators may prefer to use it for reference only.)
Cousins, J., *Make it Happy*, Penguin, 1979
(This book was written for young people, but some educators may prefer to use it for reference only.)
Docherty, Dr. J., *Growing Up: A Guide for Children and Parents*, Modus, 1986
(available from the FPA Bookshop. This book uses pictures of black people throughout.)
Keable-Elliott, D., *You and Your Body: A Complete Guide*, Hamish Hamilton, 1983
Mayle, P., *Where Did I Come From?*, Macmillan, 1978
Rayner, C., *The Body Book*, Piccolo, 1979
(for children.)
Rayner, C., *Growing Pains — And How To Avoid Them*, Corgi, 1984
Singer-Kaplan, H., *Making Sense of Sex*, Quartet 1980

### Videos/Films

Body Image
Down There
Learning to Love
Let's Talk About It: Male and Female
Sex Education: Growing, Life Begins

### Additional Resources

Fit For Life
The Grapevine Game
Life (Talking Points, Set 2)
Male and Female (FPA)
Sexuality and the Mentally Handicapped: Parts 1, 5
Think Well, Units 1, 2

### Activities

53  There's another name for it
54  Naming the parts
55  What's in the bag? — collage
56  My body
57  Clothes line or kite string
58  What I do with my body
59  Test your knowledge
60  What is sexuality?
61  What is sexual maturity?
62  What is appropriate behaviour?
63  Sexual response — Have you got an answer?

# 53 There's another name for it

| | |
|---|---|
| **Objectives** | To familiarise participants with different sexual vocabularies.<br>To illustrate that different groups are more comfortable with different terminology.<br>To illustrate cultural, social and sexual attitudes to sex revealed in language. |
| **Prerequisites** | None. |
| **Age group** | 13-16, 16 +<br>Part of this activity could be adapted for use with younger children, to establish suitable terminology. |
| **Group size** | Ideally a maximum of 25. |
| **Time needed** | 40 minutes. |
| **What you need** | Large sheets of paper, felt-tip pens for each group.<br>To have read *What language will be used?* (page 14). |

**How you do it**

a Explain to the participants that in order to communicate effectively about sex, it is important to have an understanding of both medical and common terminology. Explain that it is normal and acceptable to feel uncomfortable with certain sexual words and expressions.

b Have the large group form into groups of 3 or 4 and find themselves comfortable working spaces.

c Tell the participants that you will call out a word and they are to brainstorm (page 21) all the other words they know with similar meaning.

d When all the words have been brainstormed, re-form the large group and share the lists.

e Explore the words which may be used by:
doctors,
adults with each other,
adults with children,
young people with each other,
young children with each other,
women,
men.

f Explore the cultural, social and sexual attitudes that are revealed in the language we use.

▶ **Suggested words**
vagina
penis
masturbate
orgasm
sexual intercourse
pregnant
breasts
testes

# **54** Naming the parts

| | |
|---|---|
| **Objectives** | To identify the level of knowledge in the group about the reproductive system.<br>To provide an opportunity for group co-operation.<br>To share knowledge in a co-operative setting. |
| **Prerequisites** | Some knowledge of the reproductive system. |
| **Age group** | 13-16, 16 + |
| **Group size** | Ideally a maximum of 25. |
| **Time needed** | 20-30 minutes. |
| **What you need** | Multiple copies of the diagrams (pages 113, 114).<br>A chart with clearly defined female and male pelvic organs. |

**How you do it**

a  Have the group form into groups of 3 or 4 and find comfortable working spaces.

b  Provide each group with a copy of the diagrams.

c  Ask each group to label all the parts shown on the diagrams.

d  Share the results and have participants correct their diagrams.

**Variation**  Have the groups draw and label their own diagrams.

Female Pelvic Organs
1 Fallopian tube
2 Ovary
3 Uterus
4 Cervix
5 Vagina
6 Vaginal opening
7 Clitoris
8 Vaginal lips
9 Pubic bone
10 Pubic hair
11 Bladder
12 Urethra
13 Urethral opening
14 Rectum
15 Anus

Male Pelvic Organs
1 Penis
2 Glans
3 Foreskin
4 Bladder
5 Urethra
6 Urethral opening
7 Prostate gland
8 Seminal vesicle
9 Vas deferens
10 Epididymis
11 Testicle
12 Scrotum
13 Pubic bone
14 Pubic hair
15 Rectum
16 Anus

# Female pelvic organs

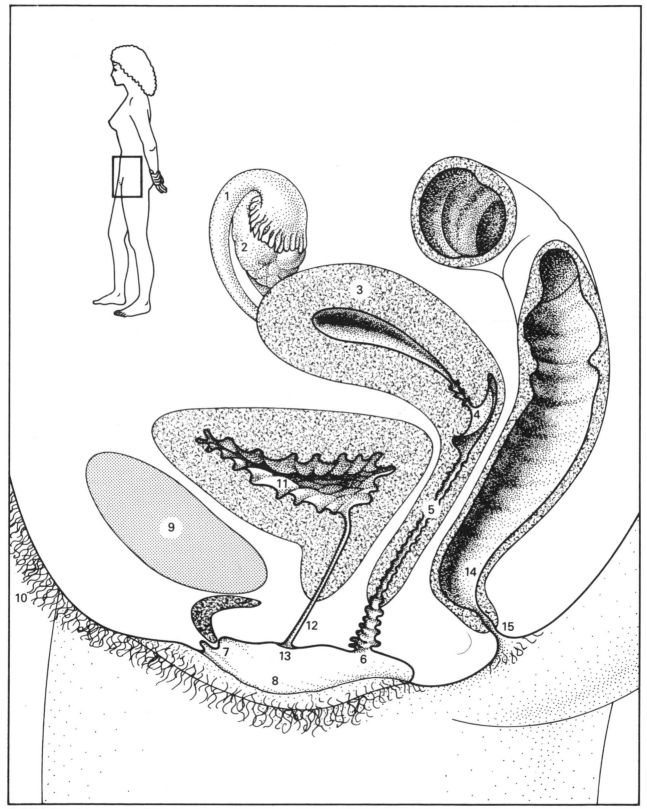

# Male pelvic organs

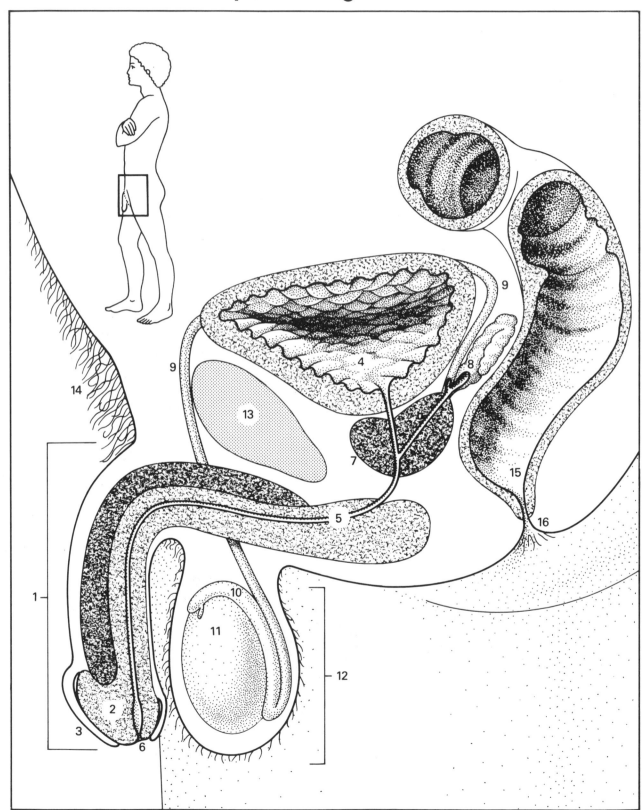

# 55 What's in the bag? - collage

| | |
|---|---|
| **Objectives** | To evaluate the participant's level of knowledge about the reproductive system.<br>To provide information about the reproductive systems in an enjoyable and practical way. |
| **Prerequisites** | Some knowledge of the reproductive system. |
| **Age group** | 9-13, 13-16, 16 + |
| **Group size** | Ideally a maximum of 25. |
| **Time needed** | 30-40 minutes. |

**What you need**　A 'mystery bag' for each individual or group containing:

| | |
|---|---|
| 1 large piece of cardboard | a piece of aluminium foil |
| 2 ping-pong balls | 2 uninflated balloons |
| string | glue |
| coloured wool | scissors |
| playdough or clay | sticky tape |
| 2 paper clips | felt-tip pen |
| pipecleaners | |

**How you do it**

a　Give each individual or group a 'mystery bag'.

b　Allocate the female OR male reproductive system to each individual or group and ask them to depict the system using the contents of the 'mystery bag'.

c　Allow time at the end of the session for showing and sharing.

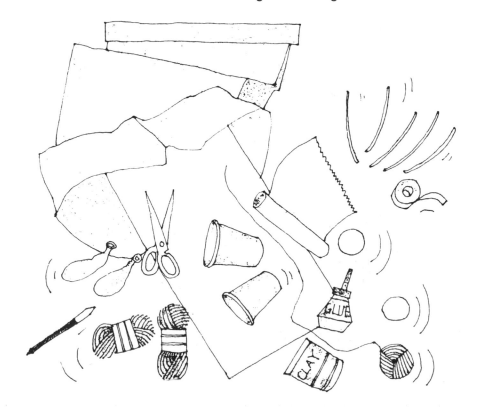

# 56 My body

**Objective**    To promote discussion on body image and self-esteem.

**Prerequisites**    None.

**Age group**    13-16, 16+

**Group size**    Ideally a maximum of 25.

**Time needed**    15 minutes.

**What you need**    A copy of the *Continuums* (page 117) for each participant.

**How do you do it**

a Hand out copies of the continuums. Stress that this activity will describe how the participants feel today and not necessarily how they might have felt in the past, or will feel in the future.

b Stress that this is a private activity.

c Ask participants to mark their positions on the continuums.

d After they have finished the continuums, ask the participants to complete a *Sentence stem* (page 34).

e In small groups share the completed sentences and allow time for discussion.

**Note**    Make up other continuums to suit the group, the subject matter, and your goals for the session.

# My body . . . continuums

Mark the point on the continuum which best describes your reaction, or how you feel.

How do you feel about your body?

......................................................................................................

totally
satisfied

totally
dissatisfied

Would you rather be?

......................................................................................................

very
strong

very
weak

I want my body to be

......................................................................................................

the thing that
people most
remember me for

the thing that
people least
remember me for

I would rather be

......................................................................................................

overweight
and fit

underweight
and unfit

© LDA taught not caught

Permission to copy this page for participant use.

# 57 Clothes line or kite string

| | |
|---|---|
| **Objectives** | To provide a starting point for a discussion on body image.<br>To encourage the participants to describe their bodies in abstract terms. |
| **Prerequisites** | Positive support in the group.<br>Literacy skills. |
| **Age group** | 13-16, 16 + |
| **Group size** | Ideally a maximum of 25. |
| **Time needed** | 30 minutes. |
| **What you need** | Paper and pen for each participant. |

**How you do it**

a  Ask the participants to think about their bodies in relation to the pairs of words which will be read out. The concepts in this activity are abstract, so ask the participants to think about the images which come to mind each time words are given, and relate the images to themselves.

b  Read out the choices, saying:
'How would you describe your body? Is it more like . . . or . . . ?'
Each pair of words is introduced with this statement.

| | | |
|---|---|---|
| moonshine | *or* | sunshine |
| solid | *or* | liquid |
| beer | *or* | champagne |
| Monday | *or* | Saturday |
| green | *or* | orange |
| velvet | *or* | cotton |
| Volkswagen | *or* | Rolls Royce |
| bunch of violets | *or* | a long stemmed rose |
| cat | *or* | dog |
| clothes line | *or* | kite string |

c  Between each pair of words allow time for the participants to write down the word that best describes their bodies.
Keep this activity flowing so that participants select the word which first comes to mind.

d  Ask the participants to reflect on their choices and write a *Sentence stem* (page 34).
Then ask them to share the results of their reflections in small groups.

**Follow-up**  Using the same pairs of words, ask the participants — 'How would you describe YOURSELF?' 'Are you more like . . . or . . . ?
Then ask them to compare the two lists and discuss any difference between the way they see their bodies and the way they see themselves.

118

# **58** What I do with my body

| | |
|---|---|
| **Objectives** | To clarify personal feelings about body image.<br>To start a process enabling participants to develop positive attitudes towards their bodies. |
| **Prerequisites** | Positive support in the group.<br>Literacy and numeracy skills. |
| **Age group** | 13-16, 16+ |
| **Group size** | Ideally a maximum of 25. |
| **Time needed** | 30 minutes. |
| **What you need** | A copy of the *Selection ladder* (page 120) for each participant. |

**How you do it**

a Hand out copies of the *Selection ladder*.

b First complete *What I need most/least* (page 120), by ranking the *5* senses in order from *1*, 'What I need most'; to *5* 'What I need least'. Then complete *What I do most/least*.
Explain that although it may be difficult, people must rank the options and place them on the ladder from *1* to *12*.
*1* being 'What I do *most* with my body', and
*12* being 'What I do *least* with my body'.
*NO* exceptions, *NO* equal rankings, *NO* omissions.

c Allow 10 minutes for completion of the ranking. Explain to participants that they may share their rankings if they choose.

d Have the participants complete *Sentence stems* (page 34) which will be shared in small groups.

e Allow an opportunity for discussion in the large group.

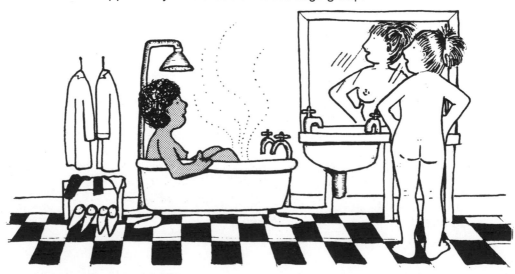

# Selection ladder

What I need most    1 ...............................................................................

2 ...............................................................................

3 ...............................................................................

4 ...............................................................................

What I need least    5 ...............................................................................

| sight | touch | taste | smell | hearing |

What I do most with    1 ...............................................................................

my body    2 ...............................................................................

3 ...............................................................................

4 ...............................................................................

5 ...............................................................................

6 ...............................................................................

7 ...............................................................................

8 ...............................................................................

9 ...............................................................................

10 ...............................................................................

11 ...............................................................................

What I do least with    12 ...............................................................................

my body

| | | |
|---|---|---|
| check it | worry about it | criticise it |
| enjoy it | touch it | care for it |
| forget about it | display it | use it |
| admire it | smell it | look at it |

Permission to copy this page for participant use.

# 59 Test your knowledge

| | |
|---|---|
| **Objectives** | To ascertain the levels of knowledge of the reproductive system in the group.<br>To provide an opportunity for participants to identify areas in which they would like more knowledge. |
| **Prerequisites** | None. |
| **Age group** | 13-16, 16 + |
| **Group size** | Any size. |
| **Time needed** | 30 minutes. |
| **What you need** | A copy of the *Question sheet* (page 122) for each participant. |

**How you do it**

a  Provide each participant with a copy of the question sheet and inform them that this is not a test to be passed or failed.

b  Ask them to write the correct term in the space provided.
Allow time for the participants to complete their question sheets.

c  Read out the correct answers and allow the participants to clarify points they did not understand.

**Note**

It may be useful for participants to discuss their answers in pairs before the educator goes through them with the whole group.

Test your knowledge — Answers

| | | | |
|---|---|---|---|
| a scrotum | f ovum | k spontaneous abortion |
| b uterus | g fallopian tubes | l erection |
| c placenta | h circumcision | m puberty |
| d semen | i ovaries | n ejaculation |
| e sperm | j testes | |

# Test your knowledge - question sheet

**Write the correct term in the space provided.**

| | | |
|---|---|---|
| uterus | ovum | puberty |
| fallopian tubes | placenta | semen |
| ovaries | sperm | circumcision |
| scrotum | spontaneous abortion | testes |
| erection | | ejaculation |

a............................... pouch containing the testicles.

b............................... pear shaped organ in the female, where the foetus grows until birth.

c............................... an organ of spongy blood cells by which the foetus is attached to the lining of the uterus, and through which the foetus is fed and its wastes are eliminated.

d............................... whitish fluid ejaculated by the male at climax, containing male sex cells.

e............................... mature reproductive cells of the male which are capable of fertilising the female ovum.

f............................... female reproductive cell, which after fertilisation begins developing into an embryo.

g............................... passages through which the ova are transported to the uterus and where fertilisation takes place.

h............................... surgical removal of the foreskin from the penis.

i............................... female reproductive glands.

j............................... male reproductive glands.

k............................... expulsion of the foetus from the uterus before it is ready to survive.

l............................... stiffening and enlargement of the penis as blood engorges the spongy tissues during sexual arousal.

m............................... period of physical change when human beings become capable of reproducing.

n............................... emission of seminal fluid.

# **60** What is sexuality?

| | |
|---|---|
| **Objectives** | To reach a working definition of the concept of sexuality.<br>To stimulate discussion and share different points of view about sexuality. |
| **Prerequisites** | None. |
| **Age group** | 16 + |
| **Group size** | Ideally a maximum of 25. |
| **Time needed** | 30-45 minutes. |
| **What you need** | Large sheets of paper, felt-tip pens, several definitions of sexuality from different reference sources. |

**How you do it**

a  Divide the group into small groups of 3 or 4, and give each group paper and a pen.

b  Ask the groups to discuss 'What is sexuality?'
Have them attempt to reach consensus about a definition.
Ask them to keep records of their discussion.

c  After 15-20 minutes re-form the large group.
Ask each group to share its definition and other important aspects of discussion, comparing similarities and differences.

d  At this point, share some of the prepared definitions of sexuality.
There are quite diverse definitions and understandings of sexuality.

e  Some important points for discussion:

the cultural constraints on our sexuality

the relationship of our self-esteem to our expressions of sexuality

the range of expressions of sexuality including celibacy, bisexuality, homosexuality and heterosexuality

the sexist and heterosexist assumptions expressed in the definitions.

# 61 What is sexual maturity?

**Objective**    To reach some understanding regarding the concept of sexual maturity.

**Prerequisites**    Participation in *What is sexuality?* (page 123).

**Age group**    16 +

**Group size**    Ideally a maximum of 25.

**Time needed**    20-30 minutes.

**What you need**    Large sheets of paper, felt-tip pens.

**How you do it**

a  Divide the group into small groups of 3 or 4.

b  Ask the small groups to discuss what they understand by the term *sexual maturity* and to record the major points of their discussion.

c  After 10-15 minutes, re-form the large group.

d  Ask each small group to share its discussion points.

e  Focus discussion on the similarities and differences in people's ideas of sexual maturity. See *What is sexuality?* point e (page 123).

# 62 What is appropriate behaviour?

| | |
|---|---|
| **Objectives** | To explore how sexuality is expressed in behaviour. |

**Objectives**

To explore how sexuality is expressed in behaviour.
To discuss the concept of appropriate and inappropriate behaviour.
To provide the opportunity for group members to clarify behaviour which is acceptable to them
To increase tolerance towards a range of expressions of sexuality.

**Prerequisites**

A feeling of trust and acceptance within the group.

**Age group**

16+

**Group size**

Ideally a maximum of 25.

**Time needed**

1 hour.

**What you need**

A set of 16 cards for each group. Each card has one situation written on it (page 126).

**How you do it**

a  Divide the group into small groups of 3 or 4.

b  Explain that the groups will be given a set of cards, each of which describes a different situation.

c  Hand out a set of cards to each group.

d  As each card is read out by a member of the small group, individuals note whether or not the situation is acceptable to them personally, and then whether or not they feel it is acceptable to the community or society.

e  The group then attempts to reach consensus on whether the behaviour is appropriate or inappropriate. Those cards designated appropriate should be placed in one pile, and those designated inappropriate in another pile. Where agreement cannot be reached, the cards are placed in a third pile. When all the situations have been assessed, the third pile is discussed in a further attempt to reach consensus. Stress that consensus does not mean forcing people to change their views.

f  Allow the groups 30 minutes to complete this part of the activity.

g  Bring the small groups back together.

h  Ask a member of one small group to read the pile of cards designated *appropriate* by her or his group. Other groups match any of their *appropriate* pile to this list. By doing this, the total group has an *appropriate* pile. Use the same procedure for *inappropriate* starting with a different small group. The remaining list of undecided or non-agreement cards can provide the start for general discussion.

i  Some questions for general discussion:
Why is certain behaviour appropriate or inappropriate?
Is age an important factor?
What do you feel if behaviour is acceptable to you but unacceptable to the community?
Have your views on these things changed over the last few years?
Do you think unacceptable behaviour should be punished?
Would you like to discuss or know more about certain situations?

# Situations

1  A fourteen year old boy is in the shower and his sister comes into the bathroom to clean her teeth. Mother comes in and tells the daughter off.

2  A young man returns from overseas. He greets the men meeting him with hugs and kisses, and shakes hands with the women.

3  A group of friends are on a beach together. The women take off their bikini tops.

4  Parents are in bed together having sexual intercourse when their three year old enters the room. They separate and then include the child in their embrace.

5  A couple are fumbling in the back seat of a car. One urges the other saying 'let's go all the way'. The other says 'no'.

6  A woman is breast feeding her baby on a bus.

7  Two women friends are walking through the park holding hands.

8  A middle aged woman and a young man are cuddling in the back row of the cinema.

9  A mother is changing her baby son's nappy. He shows by giggling, that he enjoys having his penis touched. She continues to touch him all over, including his penis.

10  Two elderly people are booked into a hotel for a pensioner's conference. They demand a room with a double bed; the clerk had reserved a twin room.

11  Two men are talking. One is obviously distressed. After some time the other has to leave and kisses his companion goodbye.

12  Two young women are being introduced. They shake hands.

13  In the office, a woman is constantly teased about the size of her breasts by the men who work with her.

14  A group of three year old children are playing doctors and patients. The boys, who are the patients show their penises to the girls who are the doctors.

15  A boy sits on his grandfather's knee. Grandfather strokes his hair.

16  A thirteen year old girl is masturbating in her room. The door is shut but not locked.

# **63** Sexual response — have you got an answer?

| | |
|---|---|
| **Objectives** | To provide correct information and rectify misconceptions regarding sexual response. |
| | To provide an opportunity for young people to ask questions that they may find difficult to ask. |
| | To provide a basis for further discussion on sexual response. |
| **Prerequisites** | None. |
| **Age group** | 16+ |
| **Group size** | Ideally a maximum of 25. |
| **Time needed** | 30-40 minutes. |
| **What you need** | *Have you got an answer?* questions (page 128) written on separate slips of paper. |
| | A shoe box, hat or similar container. |
| | A detailed knowledge of human sexual response. |

**How you do it**

a  Place the questions in the box.

b  Explain that members of the group are to draw out a piece of paper, and read the question aloud.

c  Explain that as each question is read out, you will answer. Do this accurately, and in a simple, straightforward manner.

d  When all the questions have been answered, discuss them, paying special attention to those which caused strong reactions such as concern, humour or disbelief.

**Variations**

1  Encourage members of the group to answer the questions themselves.

2  Have group members formulate their own questions and put these anonymously in the box. This method might be useful with younger age groups.

# Have you got an answer?

The references listed on the fact sheet will provide information and discussion material for these questions.

1 Is the sexual response cycle basically the same for women and men?

2 What is the function of the clitoris?

3 Is it usual for sexual stimulation to lead to sexual intercourse?

4 Where does the lubrication in the vagina come from during sexual stimulation and why is it important?

5 What happens if a man has an erection, but does not have sexual intercourse?

6 What are the phases of the sexual response cycle?

7 How do situations and feelings play a role in sexual response?

8 Is there a point in the sexual response cycle when orgasm becomes inevitable?

9 What changes take place in a woman's body during the sexual response cycle?

10 What is an orgasm?

11 What changes take place in a man's body during the sexual response cycle?

12 Do all woman have multiple orgasms, and what about men?

13 Is the sexual response cycle the same during masturbation as it is for intercourse?

14 Is simultaneous orgasm the ultimate goal of sexual intercourse?

15 Does sexual desire decrease with age?

# Puberty

### Factors to Consider
Adolescence, physical changes, emotional changes, social aspects, variation in age and length of time in which changes occur, developmental stages.

### Words the Educator May Want to Know and Understand
Acne, body hair, body shape and size, breasts, ejaculation, erection, hormones, masturbation, menarche, menstrual cycle, nocturnal emissions, puberty, internal and external reproductive organs, secondary sexual characteristics, sexual maturity, voice.

### References
Bell, R., et al., *Changing Bodies, Changing Lives*, Random House, New York, 1980

### Readings for Participants
Burkitt, A., *Learning to Live With Sex*, FPA, 1980
Mayle, P., *What's Happening to Me?*, Macmillan, 1978
Rayner, C., *Growing Pains — And How To Avoid Them*, Corgi, 1984

### Videos/Films
Am I Normal?
Growing Up — A Guide to Puberty
Learning to Love
Let's Talk About It: Puberty
Sex Education: Growing, Life Begins
Then One Year

### Additional Resources
Fit for Life
The Grapevine Game
Growing Up
Health Education, 13-18: Coming of Age
It Happens to Us All
Sample Education Pack
Sexuality and the Mentally Handicapped: Parts 2, 3
Think Well: Unit 2
Time of the Month

### Activities
64  Changes
65  When I was 13
66  I feel . . .
67  Media collage
68  Popstruck
69  Puberty quiz

# **64** Changes

**Objectives**      To involve participants in identifying both physical and emotional changes during puberty.
To encourage participants to communicate with each other about puberty.

**Prerequisites**      None.

**Age group**      9-13, 13-16, 16 +
For groups past puberty the activity becomes retrospective.

**Group size**      Ideally a maximum of 25.

**Time needed**      45 minutes.

**What you need**      Large sheets of paper, felt-tip pens, paint, fabrics, magazines.

**How you do it**

a  Divide the group into threes and give each group two pieces of paper and pens.

b  Ask each small group to draw the outline of a body large enough to fill the page.
Stress that this is not an art contest.

c  Working collectively, they are to draw in all the physical and emotional changes that occur during puberty to a male.
They may resort to using words to indicate the changes if illustrations cannot be used.

d  When they have finished the male body, ask the groups to take the other page and follow the same process for the female.

e  On completion, ask each group to share their drawings with the large group. Feed in information when necessary; clarify and discuss the changes that occur during puberty.

**Variations**

1  Divide the group into pairs. One person lies on a very large sheet of paper while the other draws around the body shape.
Using felt-tip pens, paint, fabrics, magazines and paraphernalia they then make a collage of themselves at puberty.
The small groups then share their collages with the large group, marking in any changes that they overlooked.

2  After they have drawn the body changes, ask the group to indicate with a different colour, all the changes to the body that are socially imposed such as shaving and make-up.
Follow-up with a discussion about the reasons why people make these changes.

# 65 When I was 13

| | |
|---|---|
| **Objective** | To assist participants to identify with the issues associated with puberty. |
| **Prerequisites** | None. |
| **Age group** | 16 + |
| **Group size** | Ideally a maximum of 25. |
| **Time needed** | 45 minutes. |
| **What you need** | Large sheets of paper, felt-tip pens. |
| **How you do it** | |

a Hand out paper and pens and ask participants to depict themselves graphically, symbolically or abstractly as they were when they were thirteen.
Memories can be prompted with such questions as:
What year was it?
Who was the Prime Minister?
What did you wear?
What did you most enjoy doing?
How did you feel about school?
Who was your closest friend?
Who were the most important people in your life?
What was your favourite song; activity; subject; place?
Who was your favourite film star?

b In small groups of 3 or 4, invite participants to share their drawings.

c Re-form the total group and focus discussion on the similarities and differences for young people now reaching puberty.

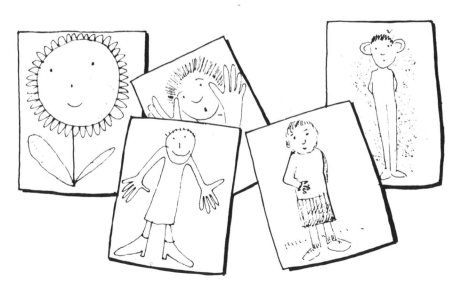

# 66 I feel . . .

| | |
|---|---|
| **Objective** | To provide an opportunity for participants to explore their feelings and attitudes related to body changes and functions during puberty. |
| **Prerequisites** | Positive support in the group. |
| **Age group** | 13-16, 16 + <br> This activity could be adapted for 9-13 year olds. |
| **Group size** | Ideally a maximum of 25. |
| **Time required** | 45-60 minutes. |
| **What you need** | A copy of *I feel . . .* (page 134) for each person. |
| **How you do it** | |

a Hand out a copy of the *I feel . . .* sheet to each participant.

b State that this is a private exercise and that there are no correct or incorrect answers.

c Tell the students that you will be reading out some unfinished sentences (see suggestions below) and they are to circle the word on their sheets that best describes their reactions to, or how they feel about, that sentence. If there is no word on the sheet to describe their feelings, they may write their own words.

d When all the sentences have been read and the participants have reacted, ask them to look at their sheets and see how many of the words that they have circled are positive and how many are negative.

e Ask them to think about this and then, using their own words complete one of the following sentences:
The words I circled make me think that .................................................
This activity makes me feel ...................................................................

**Variation**  It is possible for the sentences to be duplicated, handed out, and finished by the participants using their own words.
Be aware that everyone in the group will need to have literacy skills for this variation.

▶ **Suggested unfinished sentences**
If I saw blood on the back of a girl's dress I would feel ............................
Periods are ...........................................................................................
The first time I got my period I felt .........................................................
The first time I found out about periods I was ..........................................
Wet dreams are .....................................................................................
The idea of having a wet dream is ..........................................................
If I woke up one morning and there was a wet patch on my sheets I would
be .........................................................................................................
The idea of people touching their own genitals is ....................................
Masturbation is .....................................................................................
If I get an erection in public I feel ...........................................................
If I see a boy get an erection I feel ..........................................................

# I feel . . .

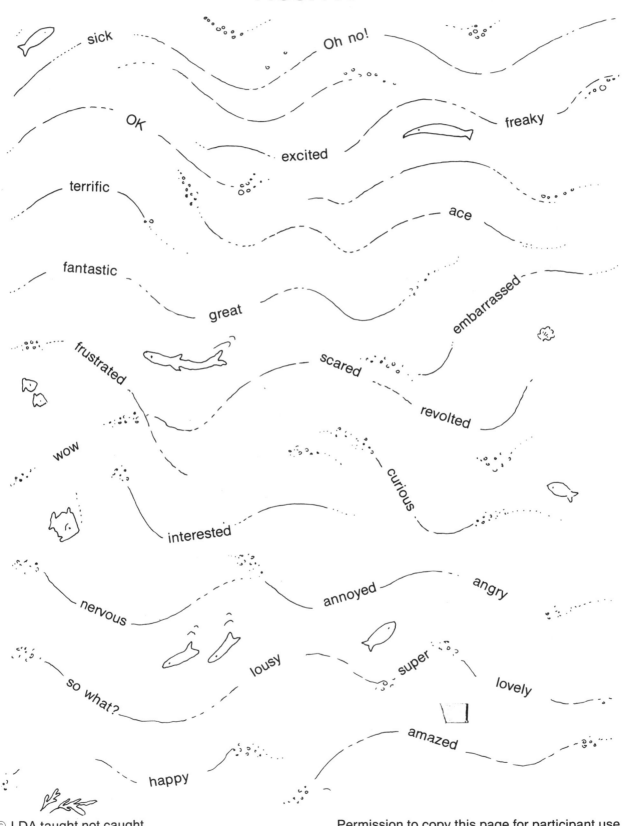

sick

Oh no!

freaky

OK

excited

terrific

ace

fantastic

great

embarrassed

frustrated

scared

revolted

wow

curious

interested

nervous

annoyed

angry

so what?

lousy

super

lovely

amazed

happy

# 67 Media collage

| | |
|---|---|
| **Objectives** | To explore the messages the media conveys about puberty and adolescence.<br>To help young people explore the influence of the media on their self image. |
| **Prerequisites** | None. |
| **Age group** | 9-13, 13-16, 16 + |
| **Group size** | Ideally a maximum of 25. |
| **Time needed** | 45 minutes. |
| **What you need** | A range of magazines and newspapers, glue, scissors, large sheets of paper, working space for small groups, display area. |

**How you do it**

a Ask the participants to work in small groups.

b Each group is to create a collage by using pictures from the magazines and newspapers which portray the media image of puberty and adolescence.

c The collages are then displayed and each group explains what they think the media says about puberty.

d Discussion points could include how realistic the images are and what effect this has on young people.

**Variation**      Collages could be made depicting the contrast between elderly and young people.

# **68** Popstruck

| | |
|---|---|
| **Objectives** | To use popular songs to encourage discussion of sexuality.<br>To explore how images portrayed in popular songs affect the behaviour of young people. |
| **Prerequisites** | None. |
| **Age group** | 13-16, 16 + |
| **Group size** | Ideally a maximum of 25. |
| **Time needed** | 30-45 minutes. |
| **What you need** | A cassette player and tapes or a record player and records. Large sheets with words of songs printed clearly and large enough for all to see. Writing material, blackboard or sheets of paper on wall. |

**How you do it**

a Tell the group that you are going to play a song.

b When the song is finished, ask each person to write, without discussion, the first two or three words that come to mind to describe the song.

c Ask group members to call out the words they have written. Write these on the blackboard or paper.

d Explain to the group that you are going to re-play the song and that you want them to listen carefully to the words.

e Play the song again, this time with the words displayed.

f Form small groups to discuss the following questions:

What is the singer saying about her or himself?

Who is she or he singing to?

What attitudes are expressed about sex, love, sexuality, marriage, the opposite sex, the same sex?

Are the words important?

Do you have the same attitudes as those expressed?

How are yours different?

Are pop and disco songs about the real world?

Are the things they sing about important to you? Why? Why not?

How do pop songs influence our personal behaviour?

# **69** Puberty quiz

**Objectives**   To identify gaps in participants' knowledge about puberty.
To allow participants to work together on finding information.

**Prerequisites**   None.

**Age group**   13-16, 16 +

**Group size**   Any size.

**Time needed**   30-45 minutes.

**What you need**   A copy of the *Puberty quiz* (page 138) and writing materials for each participant.

**How you do it**

a  Divide the large group into smaller groups of 3 or 4 and have each group find a comfortable working area.

b  Hand out a copy of the *Puberty quiz* to each participant.

c  The members of the small groups work together to answer the questions. Ensure that everyone participates in the discussion and formulation of the answers.

d  At the end of the quiz, check the responses and provide the appropriate answers. Make sure the participants mark in the corrections.

**Variations**

1  The groups could be given the list of questions and time to find the answers from books and resource people. They then present their findings to the large group.

2  Instead of distributing a copy of the quiz to the participants, write the questions on separate large sheets of paper. Display them one at a time. Read out the questions and allow time for the small groups to formulate an answer.

**Note**   It is important that quizzes are not used in a competitive manner. The references listed on the fact sheet will provide the necessary information.

Puberty quiz — Answers

| | | | |
|---|---|---|---|
| 1 | c, d | 5 | b, d |
| 2 | d | 6 | b |
| 3 | d | 7 | a, b, c |
| 4 | b | 8 | d |

# Puberty quiz

Circle the correct answer or answers to the following questions.

1   Which glands set in motion the changes in the body at puberty?
a   adrenal
b   prostate
c   pituitary
d   hypothalmus

2   The duration of puberty in the average girl is
a   2 years
b   3 years
c   6 years
d   varies considerably

3   The duration of puberty in the average boy is
a   3 years
b   4 years
c   6 years
d   varies considerably

4   Children have no sexual feelings before puberty
a   True
b   False

5   If a boy has a wet dream it means
a   he is masturbating
b   he can now be a father
c   he can control it
d   it is a way of releasing sexual tension

6   The amount of blood lost during an average period is
a   1-2 teaspoons
b   2-6 tablespoons
c   7-9 tablespoons
d   A cupful or more

7   Acne may be caused by
a   an excess of fats and sugar in the diet
b   poor hygiene
c   hormone imbalance

8   Masturbation
a   can stunt the growth
b   can lead to infertility
c   will stop you having a satisfactory sex life with a partner
d   does not have any harmful effects
e   is a sign of immaturity

# Menstruation

### Factors to Consider

Menarche and menopause, cyclic nature, hormone feedback system, myths and misconceptions, body changes, pre-menstrual tension (PMT), social aspects.

### Words the Educator May Want to Know and Understand

Amenorrhoea, dysmenorrhoea, menorrhagia, menses, menstruation, menarche, climacteric, menopause, ovary, ovulation, Mittelschmerz, primary follicle, Graafian follicle, corpus luteum, breasts, uterus, endometrium, secretory phase, proliferative phase, vagina, cervix, cervical mucus, Fallopian tubes, fimbria, cilia, pads, tampons, gonadatrophins, hypothalamus, anterior pituitary gland, luteinising hormone, oestrogen, progesterone, releasing factors, follicle stimulating hormone.

### References

Dalton, K., *Once A Month*, Fontana, 1978
Shuttle, P. and Redgrove, P., *The Wise Wound*, Penguin, 1980

### Readings for Participants

Gardner-Loulan, J., Lopez, B. and Quackenbush, M., *Period*, New Glide Publications Inc., USA: 1979
Thompson, R., *Have You Started Yet?*, Pan Books, 1987

Note: For videos and additional resources on menstruation, please see the introductory page of the section on puberty (page 129). Some reference is made to menstruation in all the audio-visual materials listed there with the exception of the film *Am I Normal?* and Part 2 of *Sexuality and the Mentally Handicapped*, both of which deal only with male puberty.

### Activities

70 'Monthly' myths and misconceptions
71 Menstrual card game
72 Period exercises
73 Keeping a menstrual chart

# 70 'Monthly' myths and misconceptions

**Objectives**    To clarify the myths and misconceptions about menstruation that exist in the community.
To separate the myths and misconceptions about menstruation from the facts.

**Prerequisites**    None.

**Age group**    9-13, 13-16, 16 +

**Group size**    Ideally a maximum of 25.

**Time needed**    30 minutes.

**What you need**    Large sheets of paper, felt-tip pens.

**How you do it**

a  Divide the large group into groups of 3 or 4.

b  Outline the rules of brainstorming (page 21). Ask the groups to brainstorm all the things that they have ever heard about menstruation, including all the myths, misconceptions, do's and don'ts.

c  Share these in the large group and make a composite list.

d  Explore the basis and origin of these myths and misconceptions, and the effect these have on our thinking about menstruation.
Clarify any questions and uncertainties.

**Variation**    Use the same technique with an older group to discuss 'How I found out about menstruation'.

**Note**    This activity can also be used for menopause or nocturnal emissions.

# **71** The menstrual card game

| | |
|---|---|
| **Objectives** | To give information about the menstrual cycle.<br>To clarify the sequence of events in the menstrual cycle. |
| **Prerequisites** | None. |
| **Age group** | 13-16, 16 + |
| **Group size** | Minimum of 15, maximum of 25. |
| **Time needed** | 45-60 minutes. |
| **What you need** | Enough space for the entire group to stand in a circle.<br>Cards 30 × 20 cm, each with one item printed in large clear lettering from a list such as this:<br>Hormones, ovary, ovum, ovulation, fallopian tubes, six and a half days, uterus, thickening of womb lining, menstrual blood/flow, 2-8 days, menstruation, cervix, vagina, sanitary towels, tampons, monthly cycle. |

**How you do it**

a Have the group sit around the edge of the room, leaving the centre clear.

b Give out all the cards.

c Say that you are going to explain the menstrual cycle and the sequence of events in the cycle.

d Tell the group that you will say the words on each card in your explanation. As each person hears her or his card named, she or he is to move into the centre of the room to form a circle which illustrates the cycle.

e At the conclusion of the explanation, all the participants with cards should be standing in the centre of the room in a circle.

f Ask the participants to explain the meaning of the word(s) on their cards starting at the beginning of the cycle and working round the circle.

g To clarify further, ask the participants to place their cards face downwards in the centre and pick up another card.

h The group is then to quickly re-form the circle in sequential order. Again ask the participants to call out the words on their cards and explain them.

**Variation**

The words can be printed on small cards and a set of cards given to groups of 3 or 4 participants. The group then places the cards in order. Reference books can be used to supplement information.

# **72** Period exercises

| | |
|---|---|
| **Objective** | To learn ways of reducing period pain. |
| **Prerequisites** | Positive support in the group, especially in mixed groups. |
| **Age group** | 13-16, 16+ |
| **Group size** | Ideally a maximum of 25. |
| **Time needed** | 20-30 minutes. |
| **What you need** | A clear comfortable floor space, comfortable clothing. |
| **How you do it** | |

a Ask each person in the group to find a clear space in the room, not too close to anyone else, in order to be able to move easily.

b Demonstrate how the exercises are to be done.

**1 Pelvic Press**
Lie flat on the floor, face down, palms on the floor beside your shoulders. Now, push your palms down on the floor, and raise your head and shoulders off the floor until your arms are outstretched. Repeat several times.

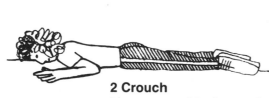

**2 Crouch**
Lie on your side, knees drawn up to your chest and head tucked under to touch your knees, in the foetal position.

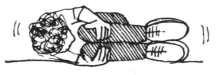

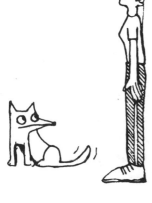

**3 Pelvic Rock**
Lie flat on the floor, face down. Stretch your arms behind you, arch your back and reach back to grasp your ankles, bending your knees and bringing your feet up to meet your hands. In this position both your legs, head and shoulders will be off the floor. Gently rock in this position.

**4 Stretching**
Stand with your back against the wall with your shoulders, heels, head and as much of your body touching the wall as possible. Try to feel as if your head is drawn upwards, making you as tall as possible. Practise this often, it is excellent for posture and for relief of period pain.

# 73 Keeping a menstrual chart

| | |
|---|---|
| **Objectives** | To help young women identify changes in feelings related to the menstrual cycle.<br>To help young women to be aware of the body changes associated with the menstrual cycle. |
| **Prerequisites** | Knowledge of menstruation. |
| **Age group** | 13-16, 16+ |
| **Group size** | Any size. |
| **Time needed** | Initially 45 minutes, then 5 minutes daily by each person. |
| **What you need** | Writing materials. |
| **How you do it** | |

a In order to establish a code, ask each participant to list the major feelings and physical changes that they have had during the last month. Include changes during menstruation. Code these.

Examples:

| | |
|---|---|
| A — achey | T — tired |
| E — energetic | D — discharge |
| G — grumpy | W — weepy |
| L — lively | P — pimples |
| Q — quiet | SB — sore breasts |
| C — cramps | LP — light period |
| H — headaches | |
| HP — heavy period | |

b Show the participants how to draw and fill in a chart using these symbols. Ask them to keep their charts over a month. Discuss the uses of such a chart and how it can lead to the understanding of the pattern of mood changes during the cycle, learning how to observe ovulation and so on.

**Note** While this strategy is particularly useful for young women, young men may participate in this activity with the co-operation of mothers, sisters or girlfriends.

# Contraception and sterilisation

### Factors to Consider
Advantages and disadvantages, availability, cost, effectiveness, groupings (barrier, behavioural, chemical, hormonal, physiological), medical procedure, mechanics of each method, misconceptions, responsibility.

### Words Educator May Want to Know and Understand
Abstention, applicator, condom, cream, diaphragm, foam, injectables, intra-uterine device (IUD), jelly, low dose, male pill, 'morning after' pill, ovulation, pessaries, pill, high dose, rhythm, spermicides, sponge, symptothermal, female sterilisation, vasectomy, withdrawal.

### References
Belfield, T. and Martins, H., *Introduction to Family Planning*, FPA, 1984
Cossey, D., *Teenage Birth Control — the Case for the Condom*, Brook Advisory Centres, 1979
Kane, P. A., *The Which Guide to Birth Control*, Consumers Association and Hodder and Stoughton, 1983

### Readings for Participants
Brook Advisory Centres, *A Look at Safe Sex*, Brook Advisory Centres Education Unit, 1979
(This booklet was designed for less able teenagers, but the Government considers it unsuitable for use in schools.)

Most of the books listed under the section 'My Body Myself' include information on contraception and sterilisation.

### Videos/Films
Birth Control: Myths and methods
Happy Family Planning
No Worries
Taking Chances

### Additional Resources
FPA Contraceptive Display Kit
FPIS Leaflets
The Grapevine Game
It's Your Life: Sex and Birth Control
Sexuality and the Mentally Handicapped: Part 6

### Activities
74  Contraceptive brainstorm
75  Design the perfect contraceptive
76  First words — birth control
77  Using the contraceptive kit
78  What's your reaction?
79  All about contraception
80  Who is responsible?
81  Contraceptive true or false quiz
82  Contraceptive methods quiz

# 74 Contraceptive brainstorm

**Objectives**     To identify all the methods of contraception known to the group.
To provide the educator with an opportunity to identify levels of
knowledge of contraception.
To dispel myths and misconceptions about contraception.

**Prerequisites**     None.

**Age group**     13-16, 16 +

**Group size**     Ideally a maximum of 25.

**Time needed**     15 minutes.

**What you need**     Large sheets of paper, felt-tip pens.

**How you do it**

a Have the large group form into groups of 3 or 4 and find comfortable
working spaces.

b Explain that each group is going to brainstorm (page 21) by listing all the
ways they have heard that will prevent a woman getting pregnant.

c Bring the groups together and make a composite list on the board.
Ask the participants to point out ineffective methods.
Explain why they are ineffective.
Add effective methods that do not appear on the list.

**Note**     In order to do this activity educators must have extensive knowledge
about contraception. The references listed on the fact sheet will provide
this knowledge.

# 75 Design the perfect contraceptive

| | |
|---|---|
| **Objectives** | To enable participants to identify the factors that need to be considered when choosing a method of contraception.<br>To provide a light-hearted introduction to contraception. |
| **Prerequisites** | None. |
| **Age group** | 16+ |
| **Group size** | Ideally a maximum of 25. |
| **Time needed** | 20-30 minutes. |
| **What you need** | Large sheets of paper, felt-tip pens. |

**How you do it**

a  Have the large group form into groups of 3 or 4 and find comfortable working spaces.

b  Explain that each group is to design the perfect contraceptive method, stressing that there are no financial, scientific or social constraints to observe. Encourage imaginative design.

c  They are then to draw and write an advertisement to describe their perfect method.

d  They then share their work with the large group.

**Follow-up**  Allocate an effective method of contraception to each group and ask them to design an advertising campaign to promote that method.

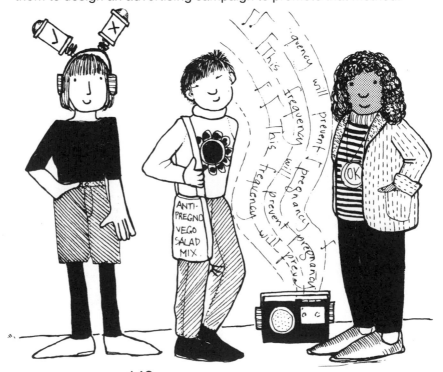

# 76 First words - birth control

**Objectives**
To enable participants to identify their feelings and attitudes about contraception and abortion.
To provide an opportunity to reflect on these attitudes.
To promote group discussion about these issues.

**Prerequisites**
None.

**Age group**
13-16, 16 +

**Group size**
Ideally a maximum of 25.

**Time needed**
30-40 minutes.

**What you need**
Pen and paper for each participant.

**How you do it**

a Explain to the participants that they will have to share with the group only as much as they choose.

b Ask the participants to write randomly on the page the first words which come to mind when they hear the word 'contraception'. Tell them to write quickly without pausing to evaluate.

c When everyone has finished, ask them to look at what they have written and circle the word or words that are most important to them. Then ask them to write a sentence which explains why those words are important.

d On the other side of the page, repeat steps b and c, substituting the word 'abortion' for 'contraception'.

e Ask the students to look at the words on the two sides of the papers noting similarities or differences, positives or negatives, areas of conflict. Then ask them to complete *Sentence stems* (page 34).

f Have the large group form into groups of 3 or 4 to share their learning.

# **77** Using the contraceptive kit

| | |
|---|---|
| **Objectives** | To enable the participants to see and handle contraceptive devices.<br>To increase familiarity with a range of contraceptive methods. |
| **Prerequisites** | Some knowledge of anatomy and physiology of the reproductive system. |
| **Age group** | 13-16, 16 + |
| **Group size** | Ideally a maximum of 25. |
| **Time needed** | 40-50 minutes. |
| **What you need** | A knowledge of all the methods of contraception.<br>A Contraceptive Kit consisting of:<br>Packets of different kinds of contraceptive pills; an intra-uterine device (IUD); a diaphragm or cap; a tube of spermicide; a packet of vaginal pessaries; two condoms; an aerosol container of contraceptive foam and an applicator; a contraceptive sponge. |

**How you do it**

a  Explain to the group that you will describe and show each method of contraception.

b  Demonstrate one method at a time, commencing with those that are less effective. If there is a device associated with the method, circulate it when you have finished describing it. Ensure that everyone has had an opportunity to ask questions and handle the device before commencing the next method.

c  Repeat this process with each contraceptive method.

d  For each method it is necessary to discuss: how it works, who takes prime responsibility, effectiveness, advantages, disadvantages, cost, and where to get it.

e  When describing how the methods work, it is necessary to be familiar with, and able to demonstrate: how to use a condom, how to put spermicidal cream or foam on a diaphragm, how an IUD is fitted and how to fill the applicator with foam.

**Variations**

1  The framework in which the information is presented can be altered to one of the following formats: device and non-device methods, reversible and non-reversible methods, female methods, male methods.

2  Divide the group into enough small groups to allocate one contraceptive method to each. Allow time for the groups to prepare and present all the information about their method based on the discussion points in step d.

**Note**  *What's your reaction?* (page 151) is useful to use in conjunction with this activity.

# 78 What's your reaction?

| | |
|---|---|
| **Objectives** | To explore the feelings that participants have about different contraceptive methods.<br>To examine the effect our feelings have on contraceptive choices and behaviour. |
| **Prerequisites** | None. |
| **Age group** | 16 + |
| **Group size** | Any size. |
| **Time needed** | 90 minutes, including presentation of *Using the contraceptive kit* (page 150). |
| **What you need** | A *Reaction sheet* (page 152) for each participant. |

**How you do it**

a  Hand out a reaction sheet to each participant.

b  Ask them to look down the list of words and mark the word that best describes their reaction to each method.

c  Repeat this process after you have presented *Using the contraceptive kit* (page 150) and ask the participants to note any changes in their reactions.

d  Repeat *Sentence stems* (page 34), and share the learning in small groups.

e  Discussion can then focus on how knowledge can alter feelings and how feelings can affect choice and use of contraceptives.

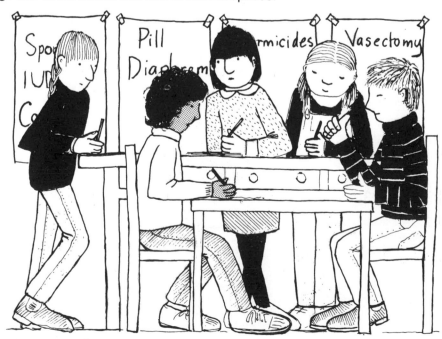

# Reaction sheet

| I think this method is: | Natural Family Planning Methods | Male Sterilisation (Vasectomy) | Female Sterilisation | IUD | Injectables | Sponge | Pill | Diaphragm/Cap | Spermicides | Condoms |
|---|---|---|---|---|---|---|---|---|---|---|
| effective | | | | | | | | | | |
| yukky | | | | | | | | | | |
| good | | | | | | | | | | |
| okay | | | | | | | | | | |
| difficult to use | | | | | | | | | | |
| not for me | | | | | | | | | | |
| messy | | | | | | | | | | |
| too permanent | | | | | | | | | | |
| medically safe | | | | | | | | | | |
| not suitable for young people | | | | | | | | | | |
| interesting | | | | | | | | | | |

# *79* All about contraception

**Objectives**
To introduce participants to the range of contraceptive methods.
To allow participants to examine the different contraceptives.
To encourage participants to collate information and present it to the larger group.

**Prerequisites**
Some knowledge of contraceptive methods.

**Age group**
13-16, 16 +

**Group size**
Ideally a maximum of 25.

**Time needed**
90 minutes.

**What you need**
A Contraceptive Kit (page 150).
Books and information on contraception, writing materials, A5 envelopes, sticky tape and cardboard box.

**How you do it**

a Put each contraceptive into an envelope — one for each group of 3 or 4 participants — seal and place it in a large cardboard box.

b Ask the large group to form into groups of 3 or 4.

c A representative from each group selects an envelope.

d Ask the small groups to list all the information they know about the selected method of contraception and all the questions they want to ask about the method.

e Each group shares the information and questions with the larger group. It is important that any inaccurate information is corrected immediately so that participants do not leave the session with wrong information.
Make sure all the questions listed in the small group are answered.

**Variation**
The small groups are given one week to find out information and answers to questions. These findings are presented to the large group.

**Note**
The educator needs a sound knowledge of all contraceptive methods to conduct this activity.

Contraception

# **80** Who is responsible?

| | |
|---|---|
| **Objectives** | To help participants identify issues related to contraceptive use.<br>To explore the concept of responsibility in sexual relationships.<br>To promote discussion about contraception and unplanned pregnancy. |
| **Prerequisites** | Literacy skills. |
| **Age group** | 16+ |
| **Group size** | Ideally a maximum of 25. |
| **Time needed** | 45 minutes. |
| **What you need** | A copy of the story *Bob and Carol, Ted and Alice and Mrs Davis* (page 103), paper and pens for each participant, large sheets of paper, felt-tip pens. |

**How you do it**

a  Give each participant a copy of the story.

b  Ask participants to read the story carefully. Then ask them to rank the characters in the story from the most responsible *1* to the least responsible *6.* Stress that there is no right or wrong answer.

c  When they have completed their rankings, ask the participants to find three or four other people to work with.

d  In the small groups they are to discuss their rankings and the reasons for their selection. At this time, participants may change their rankings if they choose.

e  Map out the rankings to illustrate the trends in the group by asking for a show of hands to indicate how many people ranked each character in each position.
For example: How many people ranked Mrs Davis number *1?*

f  Ask volunteers from the group to state which values influenced their decisions about how to rank the characters, and which criteria they used in their selections.

g  Through discussion, work towards identifying issues related to contraceptive use and unplanned pregnancy.

**Variation**

Ask the large group to brainstorm words to describe each of the characters. Discuss the differences in description.
The activity could be used to explore the issue of sexual responsibility in the light of HIV infection/AIDS.

# 81 Contraception true or false quiz

| | |
|---|---|
| **Objectives** | To check the level of knowledge of contraception in the group.<br>To provide accurate information about contraception. |
| **Prerequisites** | Literacy skills. |
| **Age group** | 13-16, 16 + |
| **Group size** | Any size. |
| **Time needed** | 30 minutes. |
| **What you need** | A copy of the *Contraception true or false quiz* (page 156) for each participant. |

**How you do it**

a Hand out copies of the quiz.

b Inform the group that this is a guide for them, not a test to be passed or failed.

c Have them answer the questions, true or false, in the spaces provided, either individually or in pairs.

d When everyone has finished, read out the correct answers and allow group members to correct their own papers.

e Discuss the answers and provide information as required.

**Variation**

Read out the questions instead of handing out the sheets.
Use arm signals. For example: hands up to indicate true, or arms folded to indicate false.

Contraception true or false quiz — Answers

1 *true* However a doctor will advise and encourage you to get your parents' consent if you are under 16. Young men do not need parental consent to buy condoms.

2 *true.* 3 *false* As far as current research shows.

4 *false.* 5 *false* This is not only ineffective, but dangerous.

6 *false* Spermicides are not 100% effective.

7 *false* This is very risky as sperm may already have been deposited in the vagina.

8 *false.* 9 *false* You may be at risk of pregnancy if you miss your Pill.

10 *true.* 11 *true.* 12 *true.* 13 *false.*

14 *false* Prevention is better than abortion every time.

15 *false* It means she is responsible — the same is true for men.

16 *false* Men have as much responsibility as women, and condoms are easy to use.

17 *false.*

# Contraception true or false quiz

Mark the answers *true* or *false*

|  |  | True | False |
|---|---|---|---|
| 1 | It is not essential to have your parents' consent to obtain contraception if you are under 16 years of age. | ........ | ........ |
| 2 | Often young women have irregular periods. | ........ | ........ |
| 3 | Taking the Pill may harm any children you may wish to have in the future. | ........ | ........ |
| 4 | Contraceptives for men are not safe or effective. | ........ | ........ |
| 5 | You can use cling film and a rubber band instead of a condom to prevent a pregnancy. | ........ | ........ |
| 6 | You can get tablets from the chemist to put into a woman's vagina which give 100% protection from pregnancy. | ........ | ........ |
| 7 | If the man 'pulls out' before he 'comes' the woman won't get pregnant. | ........ | ........ |
| 8 | Condoms — they put a hole in every 10th one. | ........ | ........ |
| 9 | If you miss a Pill every now and then, you will still be safe. | ........ | ........ |
| 10 | Correctly used, a diaphragm is an effective method of birth control. | ........ | ........ |
| 11 | It is important for any woman who is sexually active to have regular smear tests to check for cancer of the cervix. | ........ | ........ |
| 12 | If used carefully, condoms provide an effective form of birth control, and reduce the risk of sexually transmitted diseases, including HIV infection. | ........ | ........ |
| 13 | A woman can't get pregnant when she's having her period. | ........ | ........ |
| 14 | Abortion is a suitable alternative to contraception. | ........ | ........ |
| 15 | If a woman uses contraception it means she is a slag. | ........ | ........ |
| 16 | Men need not bother about contraception, that's women's business. | ........ | ........ |
| 17 | A man can feel a woman's IUD when it is in place. | ........ | ........ |

Permission to copy this page for participant use.

# 82 Contraceptive methods quiz

**Objectives**      To test knowledge of contraception.
                    To introduce accurate information about contraception.

**Prerequisites**   Literacy skills.

**Age group**       16 +

**Group size**      Ideally a maximum of 25.

**Time needed**     30-45 minutes.

**What you need**   A copy of the *Contraceptive methods quiz* (page 158) for each person.

**How you do it**

a  Hand out copies of the quiz.

b  Inform the group that the quiz is a guide for them, not a test to be passed or failed.

c  Have them answer the questions by selecting the statements they think are correct.

d  When everyone has finished, read out the correct answers and allow the group members to correct their own papers.

e  Discuss the answers and enlarge on information as required.

**Note**            Educators need to have a sound knowledge of contraceptive methods to use this activity. The references listed for this section will provide the necessary information.

Contraceptive methods quiz — Answers
It is important to be concerned with attitudes as well as information when using this quiz.
  1  b, c, d and e, a, f;
  2  b;
  3  a, b or c; the precise mechanism is still not known.
  4  i-a ii-d iii-b iv-c;
  5  i-b ii-a iii-d iv-c;
  6  b, c, d;
  7  a, c, d, e;
  8  b, c;
  9  a;
 10  b;
 11  c;
 12  d; b or c is possible depending on the woman's feelings about being sterilised.
 13  d; c is possible depending on the man's feelings about being sterilised.

# Contraceptive methods quiz

Select the correct answer or answers

1  Put these methods in order of effectiveness.
   a  natural family planning methods
   b  contraceptive pill
   c  intra-uterine device (IUD)
   d  condom
   e  diaphragm or cap and spermicides
   f  withdrawal

2  How does the combined contraceptive Pill work to prevent pregnancy?
   a  The hormones contained in the Pill kill the sperm.
   b  The hormones in the Pill prevent ovulation (the release of the ovum from the ovaries).
   c  The hormones contained in the Pill cause early miscarriage.

3  How does the Intra-uterine Device work?
   a  It prevents the sperm from entering the uterus.
   b  It stops the fertilised ovum from settling in the uterus.
   c  It immobilises the sperm.

4  Match each of the following methods with one of its advantages:

   *Method*
   i    oral contraceptive (the Pill)
   ii   The intra-uterine device (IUD)
   iii  the condom
   iv   natural family planning methods

   *Advantage*
   a  lowest failure rate if used correctly
   b  readily available without prescription
   c  no contraceptive device is used
   d  requires little attention after insertion by a doctor

5  Match each of the following methods with one of its disadvantages:

   *Method*
   i    oral contraceptive (the Pill)
   ii   the intra-uterine device (IUD)
   iii  the condom
   iv   natural family planning methods

   *Disadvantage*
   a  may be linked with pelvic infection
   b  can increase risk of thrombosis (bloodclots)
   c  awareness of the menstrual cycle is essential
   d  can interrupt the spontaneity of sexual intercourse

6  A good quality condom
   a  is not effective, even if used as directed
   b  is very effective, if used carefully
   c  gives some protection against sexually transmitted diseases
   d  can help prolong intercourse

7  The diaphragm or cap
   a  works by stopping sperm from entering the uterus
   b  has no failure rate
   c  can be obtained free after consultation with a doctor or Clinic.
   d  must be left in place for at least 6 hours after last intercourse
   e  has few side effect or dangers

8  The withdrawal method of birth control
   a  is harmful to men
   b  is the responsibility of the man
   c  does not involve chemical or mechanical devices

9  Sterilisation for a woman involves
   a  blocking or cutting the tubes which carry the ova from the ovaries
   b  the removal of the ovaries
   c  the removal of the unused ova remaining in the ovaries

10  When a man has a vasectomy (sterilisation) the operation consists of
   a  implanting a hormone in the testes which will kill the sperm
   b  blocking and removing a portion of the tubes which carry the sperm from the testes
   c  the removal of the sperm-producing section of the testes

11  When a man has had a vasectomy he can resume sexual intercourse without using a reliable method of contraception
   a  immediately
   b  after six weeks
   c  when two consecutive ejaculates have been examined and found to be free of sperm

12  When a woman has been sterilised
   a  she will not have periods any more
   b  her sex life may be improved
   c  she may be less interested in sex
   d  she will not have to worry about becoming pregnant

13  When a man has been sterilised
   a  he is unable to have an erection
   b  he will have dry orgasms
   c  his sex life may be improved
   d  his ejaculate will not contain sperm

Permission to copy this page for participant use.

# Pregnancy, birth and bonding

## Factors to Consider
Maternal changes and first signs of pregnancy, foetal development, preparation for birth and parenting, rights during pregnancy and birth, stages, choices of environment, methods of birth, breast and bottle feeding and nurturing, alternatives, cultural attitudes and customs, technological intervention, infertility.

## Words the Educator May Want to Know and Understand
Chromosomes, genes, cell division, meiosis, mitosis, multiple birth, sex determination, oestrogen, progesterone, human chorionic gonadatrophin, corpus luteum, fertilisation, conception, implantation, ectopic pregnancy, embryo, foetus, amniotic sac, amniotic fluid, chorionic villi, uterus, fundus, endometrium, cervix, dilation of cervix, labour, contractions, rupture of membranes, birth, umbilicus, afterbirth, placenta, breech, Caesarean section, amniocentesis, episiotomy, epidural, forceps, induction, oxytocin, prolactin, psychoprophylaxis, Leboyer, gestation, lactation, colostrum, in vitro fertilisation, non-sexual insemination.

## References
Boyd, C. and Sellers, L., *The British Way of Birth*, BBC That's Life Survey, Pan Books, 1982
Kitzinger, S., *The Experience of Childbirth*, Pelican, 1984
Kitzinger, S., *Pregnancy and Childbirth*, Michael Joseph, 1980
Messenger, Maire, *The Breastfeeding Book*, Century Publishing Co. Ltd, 1982
Oakley, A., *Becoming a Mother*, Martin Robertson, Oxford, 1979
Phillips, A. with Lean, N. and Jacobs, B., *Your Body, Your Baby, Your Life*, Pandora Press, 1983
Rudinger, E. (ed), *Pregnancy Month by Month*, Consumers Association, 1984
Sharpe, S., *Falling for Love: Teenage Mothers Talk*, Virago Press, 1987

## Readings for Participants
Jessel, C., *The Joy of Birth*, Methuen, 1982
Nilsson, L., *A Child is Born*, Faber and Faber, 1977 (For older children)
Nilsson, L., *How You Began*, Kestrel, 1975 (For younger children)
Writings from Hackney Reading Centre, *Every Birth It Comes Different*, Centerprise, 136 Kingsland High Street, London E8, 1980

## Videos/Films
The First Days of Life
Having a Baby: Richard's Story
Let's Talk about It: Birth Day
Sex Education: Someone New
Why Is It For Them . . . And Not Me? — Elaine's Story

## Additional Resources
Childhood
Family Lifestyles
Fit for Life
The Grapevine Game
HEC Pregnancy Book
Life Before Birth
Lifeskills Teaching Programme No. 3
Life (Talking Points, Set 2)
Sexuality and the Mentally Handicapped: Parts 5, 9
Think Well: Unit 1
What is a Family?

## Activities
83 How the body changes
84 A progressive debate
85 Media mothers and fathers
86 Breast feeding
87 Parents, families, children
88 Bill of rights

# 83 How the body changes

**Objectives**   To provide information about pregnancy.
To pool knowledge already within the group.
To stimulate further discussion about pregnancy.

**Prerequisites**   None.

**Age group**   9-13, 13-16, 16 +

**Group size**   Ideally a maximum of 25.

**Time needed**   30 minutes.

**What you need**   Large sheets of paper, felt-tip pens.
Considerable knowledge of pregnancy.

**How you do it**

a  Divide the large group into small groups.

b  Outline the rules of brainstorming (page 21), and ask the group to brainstorm all the changes that they know will occur during pregnancy, from the time of the first signs until the onset of labour.

c  After 5 to 10 minutes, re-form the large group and share the lists.

d  Discuss these, adding any changes that have not been mentioned. Clarify points and dispel myths.

**Variation**   After b, ask the small groups to draw an outline of a woman's body. Each group is to draw and mark in all the changes listed. Follow on with discussion as above.

# 84 A progressive debate

| | |
|---|---|
| **Objectives** | To examine choices and alternatives for childbirth and bonding. To raise a wide range of points on the topic in a lively, non-competitive and enjoyable way. |
| **Prerequisites** | None. |
| **Age group** | 13-16, 16+ |
| **Group size** | Ideally a maximum of 25. |
| **Time needed** | 30-45 minutes. |
| **What you need** | Nothing. |

**How you do it**

a  Choose a topic to debate (see suggestions below).

b  Form the group into two teams and allocate the for and against positions.

c  Allow twenty minutes for each team to brainstorm (page 21), and discuss the points supporting their stances. Each person in the group will be expected to speak at least once in support of the team's argument.

d  Explain to participants that they may raise new points, restate or repeat points, respond to, and refute points made by the other team.

e  Set up the room and seat participants, so that the first speakers are centrally placed and facing each other.

f  The first person in Team A presents the first point then moves. Everyone in that team moves one chair.

g  This is repeated for Team B and then continued until all the members of both teams have spoken, or the points have been exhausted.

h  At the end of this activity, it is important to help the group identify the valid and pertinent points to be considered in making decisions on these issues.

▶ **Suggested topics**

breast feeding v bottle feeding
prepared childbirth v childbirth without preparation
home birth v hospital birth
taking care of the baby yourself v hospital staff taking care of the baby
'mothering instinct' v learned parenting response

**Variations**       Use formal debating technique, Fishbowl or Hot Seat (page 20) instead of *A progressive debate*.

# 85 Media mothers and fathers

| | |
|---|---|
| **Objective** | To examine stereotypes portrayed in the popular printed media about parenthood. |
| **Prerequisites** | None. |
| **Age group** | 13-16, 16 + |
| **Group size** | Ideally a maximum of 25. |
| **Time needed** | 45 minutes. |
| **What you need** | Magazines, scissors, glue, large sheets of paper, sticky tape. |

**How you do it**

a Break into small groups.

b Provide each group with the necessary materials.

c Members of the small groups cut out magazine pictures portraying parents to compose collages. Allow 20 minutes.

d When the time is up, have the groups come together and share their collages.

e Discussion which could emerge from the collages includes:
how parent images were identified by the participants,
how often women are seen nurturing,
how often men are seen in this same role,
how the media image relates to the participant's reality.

**Variation**      Collages of mothers and fathers could be done separately to see how females and males are stereotyped in their roles.

# 86 Breast feeding

| | |
|---|---|
| **Objectives** | To introduce breast feeding as a part of the bonding process.<br>To learn about the experience from a breast feeding mother. |
| **Prerequisites** | None. |
| **Age group** | 9-13, 13-16, 16+ |
| **Group size** | Ideally a maximum of 25. |
| **Time needed** | 40-50 minutes for the actual session. |
| **What you need** | Resources requested by the speaker. |

**How you do it**

a At a time when it is appropriate to the course, explain to the group that a breast feeding counsellor from the National Childbirth Trust may be available to speak with the group. Ask for volunteers to contact the Trust in order to arrange for a counsellor, and to arrange times, dates and equipment needed.

b In a session prior to the arranged date, spend time with the group discussing the best way to use the resource person. One way of doing this is for the participants to compile a list of questions they would like answered.

c Arrange for volunteers to meet the speaker on her arrival and introduce her to the group.

d At the completion of the session a pre-arranged volunteer should thank the guest.

**Follow-up** At another session, draw together what happened during the visit and what the group learned. Relate this to the rest of the course.

# 87 Parents, families, children

| | |
|---|---|
| **Objective** | To stimulate discussion about families and relationships within them. |
| **Prerequisites** | None. |
| **Age group** | 13-16, 16+<br>This activity could be adapted for use with 9-13 year olds. |
| **Group size** | Ideally a maximum of 25. |
| **Time needed** | 40 minutes. |
| **What you need** | A copy of the statements for each group (see examples below). Pen and paper for each participant. |

**How you do it**

a  Explain that this activity is to stimulate discussion and that there is no right or wrong response.

b  Ask the group to form groups of 3 or 4.

c  Give each group a copy of the statements.

d  Ask each person in the small groups to mark their reaction to the statements in one of the following ways:
A = Agree strongly
B = Agree
C = Not sure
D = Disagree
E = Disagree strongly.

e  When they have done this ask them to share their reactions in their small groups and to talk about why they feel this way. Ask the groups to reach consensus about each statement and report back to the large group. At the end of the session the educator sums up.

f  During the small group discussions, the educator moves from group to group, so that at the end of the session, she or he can sum up the major points.

▶ **Suggested statements**
Looking after children is a woman's job.
Lots of men enjoy caring for children.
Brothers and sisters can be fun, but they can be a drag too.
Being an only child can be really nice.
People in families usually get on well.
There are many different kinds of family.
Bringing up children is hard work.
You can learn a lot from grandparents.
Families are not so important once you are older.
All men should be able to change a baby's nappy.
Working mothers show their children more love.

| | |
|---|---|
| **Follow-up** | Participants interview members of different family groupings and report back. |
| **Variation** | The statements can be written on large sheets of paper and displayed around the room. |

# **88** Bill of rights

**Objectives**

To stimulate the group to think about options during pregnancy and childbirth.
To discuss the rights of prospective and new parents during pregnancy and childbirth.

**Prerequisites**

None.

**Age group**

16 +

**Group size**

Ideally a maximum of 25.

**Time needed**

30 minutes.

**What you need**

Large sheets of paper, felt-tip pens.

**How you do it**

a  Have the large group form into small groups.

b  Ask the groups to make lists of all the aspects of pregnancy, labour, birth and the post natal time about which they would like to have some choice. Some examples could be:
choice of doctor,
use of drugs,
involvement of other people,
birth environment.

c  When the groups have finished, re-form the large group to discuss the issues.
Have the group develop a 'Bill of Rights' for new parents.

# Sexually transmitted diseases

## Factors to Consider
Signs and symptoms, sites of infection, range of diseases, transmission of diseases, frequency and incidence, where to get advice and treatment, values and attitudes, myths and misconceptions, prevention.

## Words the Educator May Want to Know and Understand
Body lice, scabies, pubic lice, crabs, Candida, Monilia, thrush, Trichomoniasis, cystitis, gonorrhoea, non-specific urethritis (NSU), non-specific vaginitis (NSV), syphilis, hepatitis, pelvic inflammatory disease, genital herpes, herpes simplex types I and II, genital warts, discharge, chancre, sterility, special clinics, genito urinary medicine (GUM) clinics, chlamydia, Acquired Immune Deficiency Syndrome (AIDS), antibody positive, Human Immuno-deficiency Virus (HIV), immune system, intravenous (IV), opportunistic infections, safer sex, virus, 'works'

## References
Adler, M. (ed.), *The ABC of AIDS*, British Medical Journal, 1987
Catterall, D., *Sexually Transmitted Diseases and VD*, Family Doctor (BMA), 1982
Chirimuuta, R. and R., *AIDS, Africa and Racism*, 1987 (available from Health-wise Bookshop, Family Planning Association)
Connor, S. and Kingman, S., *The Search for the Virus: The Scientific Discovery of AIDS and the Quest for a Cure*, Penguin, 1988
Daniels, V., *AIDS: Questions and Answers*, Cambridge Medical Books, 1986
Frontliners, *Living With AIDS: A Guide to Survival by People Living With AIDS*, Frontliners, 1987
Gordon, P. and Mitchell, L., *Safer Sex: A New Look at Sexual Pleasure*, Faber and Faber, 1988
North, B. and Crittenden, P., *Stop Herpes Now!*, Thorsons, 1983
Panos Institute, *AIDS and the Third World*, Panos Institute (new edition) 1987
Phillips, A. and Rakusen, J., *Our Bodies Ourselves*, Penguin (new edition) 1989
Richardson, D., *Women and the AIDS Crisis*, Pandora Press, 1987
Wells, N., *The AIDS Virus: Forecasting Its Impact*, Office of Health Economics, 1986

## Readings for Participants
Most of the books listed under the section *My Body Myself* include information on sexually transmitted diseases.

## Videos/Films
AIDS Help
AIDS Scene Special
Casual Encounters of the Infectious Kind (part 1)
Coming Soon
A Question of AIDS

## Additional Resources
AIDS Education for Schools
AIDS. Young Adults Project Pack
FPIS Leaflets
The Grapevine Game
Health Education, 13-18: What Would You Do . . . About Sexually Transmitted Diseases?
Sexuality and the Mentally Handicapped: Part 7
Teaching About HIV and AIDS
Teaching About STD
Working with Uncertainty

### Activities
89  First words — STDs
90  Graffiti sheets
91  They reckon that . . .
92  Getting it together
93  Chain reaction
94  Who would I turn to?
95  Where to get help — Resource File
96  STD true or false quiz
97  STD multiple choice questionnaire
98  Safer sex

# 89 First words — STD's

**Objectives**     To enable participants to identify their feelings and attitudes about sexually transmitted diseases.
To provide an opportunity to reflect on these attitudes.
To promote group discussion about related issues.

**Prerequisites**     None.

**Age group**     13-16, 16 +

**Group size**     Ideally a maximum of 25.

**Time needed**     30 minutes.

**What you need**     Pen and paper for each participant.

**How you do it**

a Ask each person to write the word 'measles' at the top of one side of the paper.

b Without discussion, have them write down all the words that come to mind when they see that word.

c When they have finished, have the group members turn the paper over, and at the top, write the word 'gonorrhoea' and all the words that come to mind relating to it.

d Ask them to compare and contrast the words on both sides of the paper, noting those in common.

e Discussion can centre around the difference in their reactions to the two words.

f Then make a comparison between gonorrhoea and measles. Include complications, sources of infections, attitudes and treatment.
Example: gonorrhoea can be cured with penicillin, whereas measles has no known treatment, only relief of symptoms.

**Variation**     The word AIDS can be substituted for the word gonorrhoea.

# **90** Graffiti sheets

| | |
|---|---|
| **Objectives** | To allow the educator to gain insight into the knowledge of and attitudes about STDs within the group.<br>To allow the participants to express their attitudes about STDs. |
| **Prerequisites** | Literacy skills. |
| **Age group** | 16 + |
| **Group size** | Ideally a maximum of 25. |
| **Time needed** | 30-45 minutes. |
| **What you need** | Large sheets of paper, felt-tip pens.<br>A sound knowledge of sexually transmitted diseases. |

**How you do it**

a Take several large sheets of paper and at the top of each one, write a different statement about STDs (see suggestions below).

b Display the pieces of paper around the room so that they can be written on.

c Have the participants move around the room and write down their responses to the statements on the paper. Encourage free expression and creative graffiti, allowing the participants to write whatever they like.

d When everyone has had an opportunity to write on every sheet, re-form the group.

e Read the graffiti and discuss such things as fiction and facts, myths and misconceptions.

**Follow-up**

This activity can be followed by further values clarification.
Example: *First words — STDs* (page 167).

**Variations**

1 Have participants form small groups and issue each group with paper and pen. The educator reads out the statements and asks the group to write their reactions.

2 Have the group form small groups and pass the graffiti sheets around for groups to write their comments.

3 Similar statements could be used, referring to HIV/AIDS.

▶ **Suggested statements**
You would know if you had an STD
Only dirty people catch STDs
You can't get an STD the first time you have intercourse.
You catch it from toilet seats.
You can get an STD more than once.
You can't have more than one STD at a time.
Condoms stop you getting STDs
Kissing spreads STDs
There's a cure for STDs

# 91 They reckon that . . .

**Objectives**     To give the educator an idea of the level of misinformation in the group.
To explode myths, and validate knowledge of sexually transmitted diseases.

**Prerequisites**     None.

**Age group**     13-16, 16 +

**Group size**     Ideally a maximum of 25.

**Time needed**     20 minutes.

**What you need**     Large sheets of paper, felt-tip pens.
Considerable knowledge of STDs to conduct this activity.

**How you do it**

a  Ask the participants to form small groups.

b  Instruct them to list all the things they have heard about STDs under the headings of true, false or uncertain.
One person should act as a recorder. Everyone should contribute.

c  After 10 minutes or when they seem to have completed their lists, bring the groups back together.

d  Have a volunteer from each group read out the list. The educator or others in the group identify the myths.

e  The educator explodes the myths and confirms the facts with supporting information.

f  Discussion of the origins of the myths is useful.

**Variation**     HIV/AIDS could be substituted for STDs.

# 92 Getting it together

| | |
|---|---|
| **Objectives** | To test knowledge of STDs after an information session.<br>To show the range of people susceptible to STDs.<br>To provide the opportunity for the group to work together to solve situational problems. |
| **Prerequisites** | An information session covering STDs. |
| **Age group** | 16 + |
| **Group size** | Maximum of 30. |
| **Time needed** | 40 minutes. |
| **What you need** | One problem or solution card from the following pages for each person. |

**How you do it**

a  Give out one card to each participant.

b  Explain that half the participants have a card that outlines a specific problem, and the other half, a card offering the solutions to these problems.

c  Group members move around the room trying to find the person who has the card which matches theirs. They ask for the information on the cards and discuss this with each other.

d  If a pair feels they are matched, they remain in the game and help others.

e  If it is obvious that some cannot find a partner, help them to do so. Then ask the pairs to sit together in a circle.

f  The pairs take it in turns to read their cards aloud. The educator should clarify and deal with issues as they arise.

**Note**

We suggest that the educator change the language of the cards to suit the group. If you want participants to have more detailed medical information on treatments, then add appropriate data.

**PROBLEM**

You hear that a girlfriend you have been going out with is an intravenous drug user. Could you get AIDS?

**SOLUTION**

It is possible if she has ever shared needles or syringes and had unprotected sexual intercourse with you. Go to a special clinic for advice.

**PROBLEM**

Your friend has stopped drinking alcohol, and everyone says it must be because he has got an STD.

**SOLUTION**

It could be he is receiving treatment for urethritis.
However, there are lots of reasons why people stop drinking.

**PROBLEM**

You are worried that the staff at the Special Clinic will want to know all about you.

**SOLUTION**

They will want to know your name and address, and medical details. However, they will not pass them on.

**PROBLEM**

You want to know where the nearest Special Clinic is.

**SOLUTION**

Lists of Special Clinics are often displayed in public lavatories. Or ask at your doctor's, a clinic or health centre. Or look in the telephone directory under 'Venereal Diseases'.

**PROBLEM**

You have noticed a genital itch and a smelly discharge that looks like cottage cheese.

**SOLUTION**

You have probably got thrush.
You should go to a Special Clinic or to your own doctor.

**PROBLEM**

The doctor says you have thrush, but how can that be true when you are not sexually active?

**SOLUTION**

It is not only passed on through sexual contact.

**PROBLEM**

You think you might have a sexually transmitted disease. What should you do?

**SOLUTION**

Go to a Special Clinic or to your own doctor.

**PROBLEM**

You are sexually active with more than one partner.
How can you minimise the risk of getting an STD?

**SOLUTION**

Suggest that you/your partner uses a condom, or practice safer sex.

**PROBLEM**

You have only ever had sex with one person. Surely you could not have caught genital herpes?

**SOLUTION**

Yes, you could, if your partner had sex with other people.

**PROBLEM**

One of your boyfriends has just told you he has gonorrhoea. He has asked you to go to the Special Clinic. What else might you need to do?

**SOLUTION**

Contact any other recent sexual partners, and suggest they go to the Special Clinic for a check up.

Permission to copy this page for participant use.

| | |
|---|---|
| **PROBLEM**<br><br>You were kissing a new boyfriend the other night, and you got a tingly feeling between your legs. It couldn't be an STD, could it? | **SOLUTION**<br><br>Unlikely. You were probably feeling sexually aroused. |
| **PROBLEM**<br><br>You have some nasty spots on your back. Your friend says it is syphilis — could it be? | **SOLUTION**<br><br>Most unlikely. You have probably got acne. |
| **PROBLEM**<br><br>You are a woman. You have an urgent need to pass urine and you feel a bit run down. You think you saw blood in your urine. | **SOLUTION**<br><br>You probably have cystitis. See your doctor and get some treatment. |
| **PROBLEM**<br><br>Last year you were treated for NSU (non specific urethritis). You seem to have a discharge again, but surely you cannot get it more than once? | **SOLUTION**<br><br>Yes you can. If you have had close sexual contact with a partner, it can recur several times. |
| **PROBLEM**<br><br>Your boyfriend says you might have gonorrhoea. You have not noticed any symptoms, so you can't have, can you? | **SOLUTION**<br><br>You could have. The symptoms often don't show in the early stages, especially in women. It would be wise to get it checked. |

Permission to copy this page for participant use.

# 93 Chain reaction

| Objectives | To clarify attitudes about STDs within the group. |
|---|---|
| | To explore the conept of responsibility in relationships. |

**Prerequisites**    None.

**Age group**    16+

**Group size**    Ideally a maximum of 25.

**Time needed**    30 minutes.

**What you need**    One copy of *Chain reaction — the story* (page 175) and writing material for each person.

**How you do it**

a  Hand out the copies of the story.

b  Have individuals follow the story as you read it aloud.
Instruct the group not to speak or comment on the story when you have finished reading.

c  When the story has been read instruct the participants to rank the characters from most responsible *1*, to least responsible *4*.

d  When people have completed their rankings, form into small groups to discuss how they ranked the characters and why.

e  In the large group discuss what different people define as responsible action and how people think the story ends. Also discuss the concept of safer sex. What could the people in the story have done to ensure that STDs were not spread?

f  A matrix can be created to show majority attitudes by totalling how many people ranked each character in the story (see below).

|  | 1 | 2 | 3 | 4 |
|---|---|---|---|---|
| Deb |  |  |  |  |
| John |  |  |  |  |
| Lisa |  |  |  |  |
| Phillip |  |  |  |  |

# Chain reaction - the story

Phillip had just returned from the doctor.
'I think you could have gonorrhoea,' said Phillip. Deb was stunned.
'But how?' she asked disbelievingly, 'I haven't noticed anything different.'

Deb and Phillip had been together for two years, and although they both had other close friends with whom they slept occasionally, it had never occurred to them that one of them could catch a sexually transmitted disease.

'You'll have to see a doctor,' said Philip, 'and if there is anyone else, tell them. My doctor says that women often don't know they have it until the infection travels right inside, so please do something quickly.' When Phillip had first noticed the burning pain and discharge from his penis, he had been worried and upset. But the doctor soon put his mind to rest, as well as relieving the pain. 'Just some tablets,' she said, 'and it should all clear up. But you must tell anyone you have slept with, or you could get re-infected and it could cause problems for them.'

Deb felt embarrassed, but she went to a Special Clinic, and the doctor there examined her and confirmed that she had gonorrhoea. 'You are lucky to have found out now,' the doctor told her. 'If it goes too long undetected, you could become sterile.' The Clinic doctor repeated the instructions Phillip had told her, and Deb left the clinic, wondering how she could break the news to John, the only other person she had slept with in the last few months.

'John, I think you might have gonorrhoea,' Deb blurted out that night. John was livid. After Deb explained the circumstances and what he would have to do, he was icy towards her and turning on her, he spat out — 'You slut, I don't want to see you ever again. How could you pass on such a vile disease? I hate you.'

Now John was really upset. He had noticed some pain and discharge, and had seen his doctor for treatment, but had decided not to tell any of his partners. He was humiliated and shy, and now he felt he had found the source of his troubles, that loose woman Deb. He was better rid of her. John also had another girlfirend, Lisa. The more he thought about the disease Deb had given him, the more he worried about Lisa. Maybe she had it too. Did that mean he could be re-infected? Perhaps she would break off with him if he told her.

Finally John plucked up courage — after all, he remembered the doctor saying he could be re-infected — and faced Lisa with the truth. 'Well, I have had a pain lately,' said Lisa, puzzled. 'Not bad pain; I thought maybe something to do with my period. Do you think it could be to do with you having gonorrhoea?' she asked. John felt cold. If Lisa had pain, maybe she had given it to him. And he had called Deb a slut and broken off with her. What was he to do?

# 94 Who would I turn to?

| | |
|---|---|
| **Objectives** | To allow the participants to think about the person they would approach in a crisis, and why. |
| **Prerequisites** | Positive support within the group. |
| **Age group** | 16+ |
| **Group size** | Ideally a maximum of 25. |
| **Time needed** | 20 minutes. |
| **What you need** | Writing materials and a copy of *Who would I turn to?* (page 177) for each participant. |

**How you do it**

a Explain that this is a private activity and that time will be given for people to share if they choose.

b Hand out a copy of the *Who would I turn to?* sheet to each participant.

c Ask the participants to write in the space provided the name of a person who fits the category in each of the boxes.

d In the space under the centre box marked 'me', participants should write how they think they would react to being told they have a sexually transmitted disease.

e They now write how each of the people they have named might react if they were told. Ask them to note positive and negative reactions.

f Ask them to select the person they might turn to if this really happened.

g Call for willing volunteers to share who they would talk to, and why they made that choice.

**Variations**

Volunteers could role-play (page 23) approaching one of the selected people.
Other situations could be used to explore the issue of support at a time of crisis.
The activity could be specifically related to HIV/AIDS.

# Who would I turn to?

older friend or relation
name:
would react

close friend of the same sex
name:
would react

me
how I'd react

parent
name:
would react

close friend of the opposite
sex
name:
would react

Permission to copy this page for participant use.

# *95* Where to get help - Resource File

| | |
|---|---|
| **Objective** | To provide opportunities for participants to gain knowledge of the resources related to STDs available in the community. |
| **Prerequisites** | Some knowledge of STDs. |
| **Age group** | 13-16, 16 + |
| **Group size** | Ideally a maximum of 25. |
| **Time needed** | 15-20 minutes. |
| **What you need** | Large sheets of paper, pens. |

**How you do it**

a  Have the participants form small groups and each appoint a recorder.

b  Allow 5-10 minutes for the groups to list all the places they can receive assistance, treatment or counselling if they think they have a sexually transmitted disease.

c  When the time is up, re-form the large group and share lists. The educator should monitor the lists for wrong or uncertain information.

d  Keep the lists as a resource file.

**Follow-up**      The group could visit or telephone agencies in the resource file to check what is available.

# 96 STD true or false quiz

**Objectives**

To check the level of knowledge in the group about sexually transmitted diseases.
To introduce information on sexually transmitted diseases.

**Prerequisites**

Literacy skills.
Some basic knowledge of sexually transmitted diseases.

**Age group**

13-16, 16 +

**Group size**

Any size.

**Time needed**

30 minutes.

**What you need**

Pens and a copy of the *STD True or false quiz* (page 180) for each person.

**How you do it**

a  Hand out copies of the quiz and inform the group that this is a guide for them, not a test to be passed or failed.

b  Have them mark the answers, true or false, in the spaces provided.

c  When everyone has finished, read out the correct answers and allow participants to correct their own papers.

d  Discuss answers, enlarging on any information and clarifying any questions.

**Note**

This is a useful activity to use following the screening of an appropriate film.

STD true or false quiz — answers
1 *true*;  2 *true*, but it will not be cured, and will continue to harm the internal organs of the body;
3 *false*, AIDS has no cure at present, nor has genital herpes; 4 *true*;
5 *false*, If you go to a Special Clinic you will be treated with complete confidentiality.
6 *false*, the chance of this happening is remote;
7 *true*;  8 *false*, some STDs can be transmitted by bodily contact;
9 *false*; 10 *true*, and you can be re-infected with a new STD while being treated for the first;
11 *true*;  12 *true*;  13 *true*.

# STD true or false quiz

Mark the answers *true* or *false*

|  |  | **True** | **False** |
|---|---|---|---|
| 1 | You can catch an STD again, even when it has been treated and cured previously. | ........ | ........ |
| 2 | Sometimes the symptoms of an STD will go away without treatment if you wait long enough. | ........ | ........ |
| 3 | All STDs can be cured. | ........ | ........ |
| 4 | Men are more likely to know if they have an STD than woman. | ........ | ........ |
| 5 | If you are under 16 and are treated at a Special Clinic for an STD your parents must be informed. | ........ | ........ |
| 6 | STDs can be transmitted through toilet seats and dirty glasses. | ........ | ........ |
| 7 | A condom will give considerable protection against STDs. | ........ | ........ |
| 8 | You have to have sexual intercourse to catch an STD. | ........ | ........ |
| 9 | Women taking the Pill are protected against STDs. | ........ | ........ |
| 10 | You can get more than one STD at the same time. | ........ | ........ |
| 11 | Women can have an STD without knowing it. | ........ | ........ |
| 12 | If you have an STD, all the people you have had sexual contact with should be informed. | ........ | ........ |
| 13 | Often the symptoms of STDs are similar to other diseases. | ........ | ........ |

Permission to copy this page for participant use.

# 97 STD multiple choice questionnaire

**Objectives**
To open discussion about the symptoms, and the importance of seeking treatment of sexually transmitted diseases.
To provide an opportunity for individuals to test their own knowledge.
To provide information about sexually transmitted diseases.

**Prerequisites**
Literacy skills.

**Age group**
16 +

**Group size**
Any size.

**Time needed**
30 minutes.

**What you need**
Pens and copy of the *STD multiple choice questionnaire* (page 182) for each participant.
A sound knowledge of sexually transmitted diseases.

**How you do it**

a  Hand out the quiz and remind the participants that STDs include all sexually transmitted diseases from syphilis and body lice to HIV/AIDS.

b  Instruct the group to complete the questionnaire.
Inform the group that this is not a test, and that no one else need see or mark the paper.

c  When everyone has finished, read out the correct answers and have each person mark her or his own paper.

d  Discussion could centre around the importance of recognising symptoms and seeking treatment, rather than trying to diagnose the disease. Also discuss prevention methods. Such as safer sex and the use of condoms (pages 183 and 184).

STD multiple choice questionnaire — answers
These answers must be expanded to cover sexually transmitted diseases adequately.
1  c;
2  d;
3  a, b (under Venereal Diseases), c, d, e, f, g;
4  a, b, c, e, g, h;
5  a, c, d, e, f;
6  b, d.

# STD multiple choice questionnaire

Circle answers you think are correct and add any comment you wish to make.

1   The most likely way to contract an STD is by           Comment:
    a  using a public lavatory
    b  kissing or touching another person
    c  having sexual intercourse with an infected person
    d  sharing utensils with other people.

2   If you think you have an STD and want to go to a Special Clinic you must:
    a  have a letter from your doctor
    b  have parental permission
    c  take an early morning urine specimen when you go
    d  do none of the above things.

3   The address of the local STD clinic is available:
    a  at a health centre
    b  in the telephone book
    c  from a local doctor
    d  from the school counsellor or nurse
    e  at the Citizen's Advice Bureau
    f  at the casualty department of the local hospital
    g  from the Family Planning Association.

4   The symptoms of STDs in women are:
    a  an unusual vaginal discharge
    b  burning when passing urine
    c  abdominal pain and painful joints
    d  longer, heavier periods than usual
    e  pain during intercourse
    f  constipation
    g  burning, itchy vagina
    h  or you can have no symptoms at all

5   The symptoms of STDs in men are:
    a  pain when passing urine
    b  constipation
    c  discharge from the penis
    d  rash on the face and the body
    e  itching in the urethra
    f  or you can have no symptoms at all.

6   If you discover that you have an STD, who of the following must be informed?
    a  your parents
    b  your sexual partners
    c  your family doctor
    d  the person who infected you

                Permission to copy this page for participant use.

# 98 Safer sex

| | |
|---|---|
| **Objectives** | To raise and discuss issues about safe sex. To raise and clarify some of the assumptions people make about AIDS. |
| **Prerequisites** | Literacy skills. |
| **Age group** | 13-16, 16 + |
| **Group size** | Any size. |
| **Time needed** | 40 minutes. |
| **What you need** | A copy of *Safer sex — the story* (page 184) for each participant. A knowledge of AIDS. |

**How you do it**

a Hand out copies of *Safer sex — the story* and ask participants not to discuss it.
Read the story aloud.

b Allow the participants time to read through and answer the accompanying questions privately.

c Invite the participants to discuss their responses either in small groups or in the large group.
Allow time to provide correct answers to questions 2-7.

Safer sex — answers
2 c, There should be no exchange of blood, semen or vaginal secretions.
a and b will also lessen your chances of acquiring AIDS.
3 d;
4 a;
5 d;
6 a;
7 a, If Les ever shared needles or syringes.

# Safer sex - the story

Les and Chris have just started a new relationship and are enjoying sharing their past experiences and stories about their lives. Chris has had a number of partners over the past few years and is hoping that this relationship with Les will be more stable and long lasting. Les has just ended a long-term relationship partly because there had been arguments about IV drug use. Les has made a conscious decision to stay clear of the drug scene in future. Chris is infertile and wonders if this will make any difference to their relationship if Les knows. Chris is also really concerned about AIDS, as there has been a lot of media coverage recently, but doesn't know how to raise the issue with Les or how to suggest that they might take some precautions and practise safer sex.

1   How might Les react if Chris raises the issue of safer sex?

2   What is safer sex?
   a   Having a mutually exclusive life-long sexual relationship.
   b   Not having a sexual relationship.
   c   Using a condom every time you have sex.
   d   Sexual activities which do not include penetrative sex.

3   Who can get AIDS?
   a   Gay men
   b   Babies born to IV drug-using mothers
   c   People with haemophilia
   d   Anyone

4   When properly used, condoms can protect you from infection with HIV (the AIDS virus).
   a   True
   b   False

5   Which of these activities might expose you to HIV (the AIDS virus)?
   a   Hugging and kissing
   b   Eating in a restaurant that employs a gay waiter
   c   Using a public toilet
   d   Sharing someone else's works when using drugs

6   As Chris is infertile, does Les need to worry about AIDS?
   a   Yes
   b   No        Why? ..........................................................................................

7   If Les has been an IV drug user, does Chris need to worry about the possibility of getting AIDS?
   a   Yes
   b   N o       Why? ..........................................................................................

**Part D**
# Reference section

# Educators, please note

The books and resources listed here are only a selection of those available.

* It is essential that you preview all A/V materials to decide whether they are suitable for your group. Synopses can be misleading, resources date quickly, and not all the items listed adequately reflect the multi-cultural nature and diverse religious beliefs of our society.

* Age ranges have been given for guidance only; after previewing, you may decide that they are not appropriate for your group.

* In the list of Videos and Films, the supplier given is the loan source unless otherwise stated. In the list of Additional Resources, however, most of the items must be purchased rather than hired. No prices are given as these change so frequently. Suppliers' addresses can be found within Useful Addresses.

* Try your local Health Education Unit or Teachers' Centre for preview or loan copies of the A/V items listed. Many of the A/V resources can be previewed at the Health Education Authority's Resource Centre, 71-75 New Oxford Street, London WC1A 1AH during office hours (9am to 5pm Tuesday to Friday) but cannot be borrowed from them, as their audio-visual collection is strictly for reference only. A selection of the books listed can be found in the Library of the International Planned Parenthood Federation, and many can be purchased from the specialist bookshops listed in the Useful Addresses section of this book.

* BBC and ITV educational broadcasts dealing with aspects of relationships and sexuality may also prove useful for those of you working in schools or colleges where there is access to a video recorder. These can be recorded off-air by holders of the relevant licence(s), and can provide a useful source of additional material.

We welcome suggestions for new materials for inclusion in our lists. Please write to the editors c/o LDA.

# Recommended Reading

Applebaum, R. L., et al, *The Process of Grouping Communications*, Science Research Associates Inc., USA, 1979

A useful book which applies the theories and research on group dynamics and communication to practical situations. Some of the areas covered are groups, communication, leadership, conflict, problem-solving, discussion methods and small group techniques.

Bell, Ruth et al., *Changing Bodies, Changing Lives*, Random House, New York, 1980

Written by members of the Boston Women's Health Collective and the Teen Book Project, this book is for teenagers, parents and teachers. It focuses on issues of concern to young people, as expressed by them, provides information about sex and body development and allows young people to hear from others who are going through similar changes and experiences.

Carrera, M., *Sex: The Facts, The Acts and Your Feelings*, Crown Publishers Inc., New York, 1981.

A comprehensive, factual book on sex and sexuality, Carrera treats sexuality within the context of the whole person, discussing the roles of relationships, age, social values and religious convictions in relation to overall sexual development.

Jackson, Stevi, *Childhood and Sexuality*, Basil Blackwell Publisher Ltd, Oxford, 1982

Stevi Jackson explores the fears and anxieties of adults about providing children and young people with information about sex. Her straightforward and honest approach raises questions for all educators of young people. She particularly addresses assumptions about the different attitudes to girls and boys and the disadvantages girls face in trying to obtain information about their sexuality.

Massey, D., *School Sex Education: Why, What and How?*, FPA Education Unit, 1988

This is a practical guide for teachers, which explores some of the issues relevant to sex education in schools today. It includes sections which will help teachers just starting sex education, those working in primary schools or special education. It also has sections on the legal situation, forming a policy, resources, teacher training and governor workshops.

Phillips, A. and Rakusen, J., *Our Bodies, Ourselves*, Penguin (new edition) 1989.

Written by, and for women so that women will have greater understanding of sexuality, reproduction, relationships, sexually transmitted diseases, birth control, abortion, parenthood, childbearing and menopause.

Spender, Dale, *Man Made Language*, Routledge and Kegan Paul, London, 1981

A valuable reference which explains the importance of language and its power to control. Of particular relevance is the section on 'naming' which explores the problems of terminology for sexuality.

Zilbergeld, B., *Men and Sex*, Fontana, 1979

An informative and reassuring book for men. Its aim is to help the reader evaluate his sexual values, feelings and preferences, to come to terms with reality and to enjoy himself.

# Videos and Films (in alphabetical order)

**Title:** AIDS HELP

**Production details:** Video. Colour. 5 × 10 minute episodes, 4 × 5 minute episodes.
ITV and Thames Television, 1987

**Synopsis:** A series of short programmes which look at various aspects of AIDS and how it affects different groups of people. On the whole the information is accurate and well-presented although rather London-based. The language is straightforward and could cause offence but what is being offered is important advice and promotion of the 'safer sex' message to both heterosexual and homosexual men and women.
Not suitable for younger teenagers.

**Distributed by:** Guild, Sound and Vision

**Title:** AIDS Scene Special

**Production details:** Video. Colour. 20 mins.
Central Television, 1987

**Synopsis:** Four 5 minute units, each consisting of an acted scene with accompanying comments by a range of people, including young adults, agony aunts and uncles. The scenes depict young people in 'real life' situations where issues arise about sexual relationships, social and peer pressure, HIV transmission and safer sex. Good for discussion.

**Distributed by:** Central Television

**Title:** AM I NORMAL?

**Production details:** 16mm, video. Colour. 23 mins. American.
Boston Family Planning Project, 1979

**Synopsis:** This film attempts to provide, in a humorous way, reassurance to pubertal boys on masturbation, wet dreams, erections, penis size etc. Some genuinely funny moments but the style of presentation, particularly in the last few scenes, might seem rather exaggerated to a British audience. Notes accompany. Age range 11 + .

**Distributed by:** Concord Films Council Ltd.

**Title:** BIRTH CONTROL: MYTHS AND METHODS

**Production details:** Video. Colour. 26 mins.
Churchill Films, U.S.A.

**Synopsis:** An American video in which common myths about sex and contraception are set against straightforward facts about current methods of birth control. The video emphasises that not having sex is perfectly acceptable and features young men and women from a variety of ethnic groups. Follow-up work on national and local family planning services in the U.K. would enhance the information content.
Age range 15 + .

**Distributed by:** Boulton-Hawker Films Ltd.

**Title:** BODY IMAGE

**Production details:** 16mm, video. Colour. 27 mins.
Thames Television, 1983

**Synopsis:** An exploration of how the mass media has helped to perpetuate the myth of 'the ideal woman'. For a model posing for a pin-up photo in a daily newspaper her body is her means of survival, while for many other women, the image she creates is an insult and a threat. Suitable for older students and women's groups.

**Distributed by:** Concord Films Council Ltd.

# Videos and Films

**Title:** **CASUAL ENCOUNTERS OF THE INFECTIOUS KIND, Part 1.**

**Production details:** 16mm. Colour. Part 1: 25 mins.
Boulton-Hawker and Oxford A.H.A., 1979

**Synopsis:** Part 1: The Facts About Sexually Transmitted Diseases.
A factual film which looks at the causes, symptoms and cures of the main sexually transmitted infections. Animated sequences are intercut with simulated interviews in which young adults attending a clinic relate their own experience of STDs. Age range 15 + .

**Distributed by:** Concord Films Council Ltd.
National Audio-Visual Aids Library

**Title:** **COMING SOON**

**Production details:** Video. Colour. 5 x 10 minute programmes. Cartoon booklet accompanies.
Central Independent Television, 1987

**Synopsis:** All five programmes are based round a discussion in a Nottinghamshire coffee bar between a culturally diverse group of young people. Strongly held views are expressed by some and attacked by others and the discussion is broken up in the first two programmes by information and anecdotes from experts and well-known personalities. But following the arrival of a man with HIV and a woman with AIDS there is a stunning change of mood with concern, sympathy and anger to the fore, although not all prejudices appear. A powerful series of triggers which need careful previewing in order to derive maximum benefit from the many diverse opinions expressed.

**Distributed by:** Guild, Sound and Vision

**Title:** **DANNY'S BIG NIGHT**

**Production details:** Video. Colour. 25 mins.
Newsreel Collective for FPA, 1985

**Synopsis:** Danny has decided that tonight is 'the big night' when he will 'go all the way' with his girlfriend Lorraine. However, the evening does not go according to plan, and ends with Lorraine storming out after Danny finds a packet of condoms in her handbag and accuses her of being 'a slag'. Made before carrying condoms for safer sex equalled being sexually responsible, but the video's original aim of encouraging teenage boys to discuss how they see themselves in relation to each other and to the opposite sex still holds good.

**Distributed by:** FPA Education Unit
Concord Films Council Ltd.
Albany Video

**Title:** **DEVELOPMENTAL WORK WITH TUTORIAL GROUPS**

**Production details:** Video. Colour. 57 mins.
ILEA Learning Materials Service, 1980-2

**Synopsis:** An observational video which shows two teachers working with second-year pupils in a London secondary school. The teachers are using an approach to tutorial work developed by Dr Leslie Button which encourages structured and sequential opportunities for personal development and group support. Of interest to any educator who is unsure about using participatory methods, or about planning and evaluating lessons in which process and content are of equal importance. Notes accompany.

**Distributed by:** CFL Vision
ILEA Learning Resources Branch

# Videos and Films

**Title:** **DOWN THERE**

**Production details:** Video. Colour. 23 mins.
Film Australia, 1985

**Synopsis:** Using a combination of animated drawings and interviews with women from many cultural backgrounds, this Australian video presents information about women's bodies and how they work in an open and positive way. Most of the main events in a woman's health career are discussed from menstruation to the menopause, and health clinics, internal examinations, vaginal infections, pre-menstrual syndrome, contraception, cervical smears and breast self-examination are looked at in some detail (note that routine smear tests are not carried out annually here as they appear to be in Australia). A warm and honest portrayal of women's bodies as they really are. For older teenagers, particularly young women.

**Distributed by:** Educational Media International

**Title:** **FEELING YES, FEELING NO**

**Production details:** 16mm, video. Colour. Four films; total running time 1 hour 11 mins. Canadian. National Film Board of Canada, 1984

**Synopsis:** A series of four films, aimed at any educator concerned about the prevention of sexual abuse of children.

The Adult Film (27 mins.)
This film discusses the nature and scope of child sexual abuse. It also introduces the prevention programme which forms the basis of Films 1, 2 and 3, showing filmed excerpts of the Green Thumb Theatre Group in action in the classroom.

Film 1 (14 mins.)
Using role-play and drama, the actors teach children to identify and communicate their good ('yes') and bad ('no') feelings.

Film 2 (14 mins.)
The actors move on to the meaning of sexual abuse, and encourage the children to assess strangers, as not all of them are dangerous.

Film 3 (16 mins.)
This film moves on to sexual abuse by family members or other trusted persons. The children are taught that they have a right to make decisions regarding their own bodies, that they can say no, and that they can and must persist in seeking help.

Films 1, 2 and 3 are designed for use with 6-12 year old children. Educators in this country might prefer to preview all four films, and use them with colleagues as a discussion-starter about how to approach this extremely sensitive, yet important, topic in the classroom. Support material accompanies.

**Distributed by:** Educational Media International

**Title:** **THE FIRST DAYS OF LIFE (English Version)**

**Production details:** 16mm, video. Colour. 22 mins.
Les Films du Levant with Guigoz-France, 1972

**Synopsis:** A powerful film which shows the growth and development of the human embryo, from the time of conception onwards, using photographic sequences of life inside the mother's womb. The film ends with the birth of the baby. Responses to the film vary; some groups, particularly girls, have been known to find the bloodiness of the birth and the passivity of the mother quite disturbing. Age range 14 + .

**Distributed by:** Boulton-Hawker Films Ltd.
Concord Films Council Ltd.
National Audio-Visual Aids Library

# Videos and Films

**Title:** **FOR BETTER FOR WORSE**

**Production details:** 16mm, video. Colour. 21 mins. Australian.
Tasmanian Film Corporation, 1978.

**Synopsis:** A married couple's relationship seems to be turning sour. They frequently fail to communicate their worries to each other, so that misunderstandings and problems continue to affect all aspects of their relationship, including sex. A final supreme effort to patch up their difficulties sets them back at square one. This film moves the focus away from teenagers to young adults, but could nevertheless be used to raise important points for discussion about marriage and long-term relationships. Australian accents may cause some difficulty. Age range 16 + .

**Distributed by:** Edward Patterson Associates Ltd.


**Title:** **FRAMED YOUTH — REVENGE OF THE TEENAGE PERVERTS**

**Production details:** Video. Colour. 50 mins.
Lesbian and Gay Youth Project, 1983

**Synopsis:** A film in which a group of lesbian and gay young people talk openly about their relationships with friends and family, their sexuality, and the oppression and discrimination they face. Good in parts, but too long, and needs careful previewing before use as some of the references to sexual behaviour and pleasure may be inappropriate for certain audiences. Intended to raise awareness, the film presents positive images of lesbian and gay people, but may also reinforce stereotyping by focusing on a group who have deliberately isolated themselves from the community. Age range 16 + .

**Distributed by:** Albany Video


**Title:** **GIRLS TALK**

**Production details:** Video. Colour. 15 mins.
Connexions, 1984

**Synopsis:** A video made by a group of 16-20 year old girls which raises questions about how far anti-sexist practice by youth and community workers and women's groups actually affects the lives and expectations of working class girls. The video explores responses to a local survey of 50 young people, and looks at media images of women, the employment scene, and emotional and sexual expectations of both sexes. An honest and open-ended attempt to raise sexism as a topic for group discussion in youth clubs, life and social skills courses etc. with girls only or mixed groups. Support material accompanies.

**Distributed by:** For purchase only from Connexions.


**Title:** **GIVE US A SMILE**

**Production details:** 16mm, video. Colour. 13 mins.
Leeds Animation Workshop, 1983

**Synopsis:** An animated cartoon combined with live action which shows, from one woman's point of view, the constant harassment to which so many women are subjected in their daily lives. This harassment ranges from verbal abuse through media stereotyping to actual physical violence, but in this film the women fight back! Suitable for older teenagers and women's groups.

**Distributed by:** Albany Video
Glenbuck Films Ltd.
Concord Films Council Ltd.

# Videos and Films

**Title:** **GREGORY'S GIRL**

**Production details:** 16mm, video. Colour. 91 mins.
Lake Film Productions, 1981

**Synopsis:** Delightful, if whimsical, full-length comedy in which Gregory, a 16 year-old schoolboy, falls hopelessly in love with Dorothy, the girl who replaces him in the football team. Eventually he plucks up the courage to ask her out, but the evening does not go according to plan . . . Given an 'A' (now PG) rating in the cinema, the film is for entertainment rather than for serious educational use, but might prove a light-hearted addition to planned work on sex roles or boy-girl relationships.

**Distributed by:** Glenbuck Films Ltd.

**Title:** **GROWING UP — A GUIDE TO PUBERTY**

**Production details:** Video. Colour. 12 mins.
John Halas for Bounty Vision Ltd., 1984

**Synopsis:** An animated film about the physiological and emotional changes which take place during puberty. The drawings are clear and attractively sequenced, and the film contains much helpful information for both boys and girls. Age range 10 + .

**Distributed by:** For purchase only from
Bounty Vision
Graves Medical Audio-visual Library

**Title:** **HAPPY FAMILY PLANNING**

**Production details:** 16mm, video. Colour. 8 mins.
Planned Parenthood Federation of America, 1970

**Synopsis:** An animated cartoon with the message that families can be planned. A couple with a young child go in turn to their doctor for contraceptive advice and reassurance. Extremely simplistic, but could perhaps be used as an introduction to the subject for some teenagers. There is no speech or commentary, but the different forms of contraception are labelled in five different languages. Age range 14 + .

**Distributed by:** Concord Films Council Ltd.

**Title:** **HAVING A BABY: RICHARD'S STORY**
(Part 3 of a series)

**Production details:** 16mm, video. Colour. 7 mins.
Health Education Authority, 1980

**Synopsis:** Childbirth from the father's point of view. Richard, present at the induced birth of his second daughter, provides the commentary for the film, and we see the positive support he is able to offer during the birth. Useful for mixed groups. Notes accompany. Age range 14 + .

**Distributed by:** Concord Films Council Ltd.
CFL Vision } Free loan

**Title:** **HOMOSEXUALITY — WHAT ABOUT McBRIDE?**

**Production details:** 16mm. Colour. 10 mins. American.
McGraw Hill Films, 1974

**Synopsis:** This film shows two boys discussing which friends they want to invite on a boating trip. When John asks, 'What about McBride?', Ben is adamantly against the idea as he thinks McBride is a homosexual. In a brief sequence following the film, Beau Bridges points up some of the main areas for discussion. Age range 16 + .

**Distributed by:** Concord Films Council Ltd.

# Videos and Films

**Title:** **IF ONLY WE'D KNOWN**

**Production details:** 16mm, video. Colour. 3 films; total running time 23 mins.
Health Education Authority and Spastics Society, 1979

**Synopsis:** A series of three trigger films for young people designed to stimulate discussion about the myths surrounding pregnancy and ante-natal care. It is essential that each film is accompanied by discussion, as some of the 'advice' given is deliberately incorrect. Notes accompany. Age range 15 + .
Part 1: Debbie and Linda (Trigger: 8 mins. Documentary: 5 mins.)
Debbie is 16 and still at school. She thinks she is pregnant, and turns to her friend Linda for help. This episode is followed by a documentary sequence between a GP and a pregnant girl.
Part 2: Clinic Talk (6 mins.)
Debbie visits the clinic and meets Sarah. They discuss ante-natal care.
Part 3: Sarah and Eric (4 mins.)
Sarah's husband Eric tries to persuade her to disregard the advice given to her at the ante-natal clinic.

**Distributed by:** Concord Films Council Ltd. ⎫
CFL Vision ⎬ Free loan

**Title:** **THE IMPOSSIBLE DREAM**

**Production details:** 16mm. Colour. 8 mins.
United Nations, 1984

**Synopsis:** Humorous short cartoon in which a working wife and mother dreams of a world where household tasks are more evenly distributed between men and women, boys and girls — an impossible dream? Nicely animated; could be used in a non-threatening way with a wide range of groups.

**Distributed by:** Concord Films Council Ltd.

**Title:** **I, MYSELF series: SEAN AND JOEL**

**Production details:** 16mm, video. Colour. 9 mins. Australian.
Film Australia, 1982

**Synopsis:** Short trigger film in which we see two young brothers trying to cope with their parents' divorce. Their father has remarried, while they have stayed with their mother, and their comments on the situation are both touching and revealing. Could be used to raise this difficult and sensitive subject with younger children, but not without adequate preparation and discussion time. Age range 9-12.

**Distributed by:** Educational Media International

**Title:** **I, MYSELF series: TRACEY AND TREVOR**

**Production details:** 16mm, video. Colour. 9 mins. Australian.
Film Australia, 1982

**Synopsis:** Short trigger film for younger children in which Tracey and Trevor discuss their reactions to traditional sex roles and to the expectations which society, their friends and family place on them as a girl and boy. The children's personal thoughts and experiences are presented without comment in order to stimulate discussion, although strong Australian accents mean that it is not always easy to catch everything they say. Age range 9-12.

**Distributed by:** Educational Media International

194

# Videos and Films

**Title:** **IT'S SEX NEXT WEEK**

**Production details:** Video. Colour. 30 mins.

**Synopsis:** Originally shown as a designated educational broadcast on ITV, this video takes a quiet, unsensational look at sex education in a Hampshire junior school and gives an airing to the views of teachers, parents, governors and pupils. Could provide a useful stimulus for discussion to primary schools wishing to consider their role as sex educators.

**Distributed by:** Central Independent Television

**Title:** **KIDS CAN SAY NO!**

**Production details:** Video. Colour. 20 mins.
Rolf Harris Video Ltd., 1985

**Synopsis:** A video for 5-11 year olds aimed at preventing child sexual abuse. Children talk to Rolf Harris about the touches they like, and about the 'no' feelings which they experience when touched in a way they do not like. Four abusive incidents are acted, ranging from approaches by strangers to sexual advances by the father, and the children talk about what to do — say no, get away fast, and tell someone you trust. The video comes with teaching notes and two books — 'Preventing Child Sexual Assault' by Michele Elliott and 'Sexual Abuse within the Family' by the CIBA Foundation — asterisks appear at the bottom of the screen when suitable points to break for discussion occur.

**Distributed by:** Concord Film Council Ltd.
CFL Vision
Rolf Harris Video Ltd. (purchase only)

**Title:** **LEARNING TO LOVE**

**Production details:** Video. Colour. 55 mins.
Mirror Vision Productions, 1980

**Synopsis:** Designed for parents to use at home with their children. A very comprehensive video which touches on most aspects of sex education (what language to use, changes at puberty, love and sex, virginity, intercourse, pregnancy, birth control, STDs, homosexuality and boy/girl relationships) in a frank and straightforward way. The presenter is Marje Proops. In the film, factual information is interspersed with discussion by London teenagers. Age range 15 + .

**Distributed by:** For purchase only from Mirror Vision Video

**Title:** **LET'S TALK ABOUT IT series**

**Production details:** 16mm, video. Colour. 5 films in series; total running time 1 hour 45 mins.
Film Australia, 1981-2

**Synopsis:** An excellent series of films, which follow through an Australian upper-primary school class (11 and 12 year olds) as they learn about human reproduction and sexuality. Should prompt much valuable discussion amongst teachers and parents about the nature and purpose of sex education in schools.
Male and Female (22 mins.)
   After a hesitant start, the children (and teachers) grow in confidence and understanding as they look into how and why males differ from females.
Birth Day (28 mins.)
   Learning about pregnancy and childbirth from a wide variety of sources. The evident interest and increasing capabilities of the children are beautifully captured in this film.
Puberty (18 mins.)
   Some interesting ways of approaching the subject of puberty with a mixed group of children.

# Videos and Films

The Teachers (20 mins.)
> The two teachers involved in the project talk about what they and the children have gained from it, and about some of the difficulties they experienced. They also answer criticisms about their 'ideal situation' i.e. two teachers to seventeen children, a pleasant classroom, and a non-disruptive group.

Parents (17 mins.)
> 9 months after the films were made, some parents were interviewed about their reactions to the project. All supported the work done in spite of their initial uncertainties about sex education.

**Distributed by:** Educational Media International

| | |
|---|---|
| **Title:** | **LIKE OTHER PEOPLE** |
| **Production details:** | 16mm, video. Colour. 37 mins<br>Kestrel Films for Mental Health Film Council, 1972 |
| **Synopsis:** | A deeply moving film which explores the emotional, sexual and social needs of the physically disabled. The two central characters, Margaret and Willie, are spastics who live in a residential home. Their plea is for society to recognise that they are just like other people in what they offer life, and in what they want from it. Age range 16 + . |
| **Distributed by:** | Concord Films Council Ltd. |

| | |
|---|---|
| **Title:** | **LOVING AND CARING** |
| **Production details:** | 16mm, video. Colour. 5 films; total running time 35 mins.<br>Health Education Authority and Family Planning Association, 1978 |
| **Synopsis:** | A series of five trigger films intended to stimulate discussion about boy/girl relationships. Age range 14 + . |

Part 1: Boy and Girl (5 mins.)
> After going out for three months together, Simon wants Sandra to have a sexual relationship. Sandra feels that she is not ready, but finds it hard to explain why.

Part 2: Boys Talking (8 mins.)
> Simon, Brian and friends chat in the youth club. Brian boasts about his latest exploits, and tries to goad Simon into talking about his relationship with Sandra.

Part 3: Girls Talking (8 mins.)
> Again in the youth club, Sandra broods about saying no to Simon. Her friends Jo and Claire have opposing views on pre-marital sex, and the discussion becomes heated.

Part 4: Mother and Daughter (8 mins.)
> Sandra's mother is worried about her daughter's relationship with Simon. Their discussion turns into confrontation.

Part 5: Parents' Talk (6 mins.)
> Sandra's parents bump into Brian's parents in a local club. Their discussion highlights differences in the way parents treat sons and daughters.

The films are designed to be used individually and must be followed by discussion. A little dated now in style. Notes accompany.

**Distributed by:** Concord Films Council Ltd. } Free loan
CFL Vision

# Videos and Films

**Title:** **NO WORRIES**

**Production details:** Video. Colour. 21 mins.
Holmes Productions, 1988, for Durex Contraception Information Service.
Optional A4 ringbound pack of teacher's notes plus trigger and information cards for classroom use can be purchased separately.

**Synopsis:** A useful video about relationships and contraception which combines dramatised sequences with animation and information presented by advice columnist, Melanie McFadycan and Dr. Graham Bickley, a family planning doctor. The message is that you can say no to sex but if you are involved in a sexual relationship it is important to 'be prepared' and to 'love carefully'. The content and style of the video have been skillfully designed to appeal to young people and the optional teaching pack helps to round off a professional and up-to-date resource.

**Distributed by:** Guild, Sound and Vision (video plus pack).
Durex Contraception Information Service (pack only).

**Title:** **1 in 44**

**Production details:** Video. Colour. 20 mins.
Nottingham Youth Theatre, 1983

**Synopsis:** '1 in 44 sixteen year old girls gets pregnant' — hence the title. This video has no story-line, but the situations and attitudes explored should provide many starting points for discussion. Age range 15 + .

**Distributed by:** Albany Video

**Title:** **PEEGE**

**Production details:** 16mm, video. Colour. 28 mins. American.
Phoenix Films Inc., 1973

**Synopsis:** In this film, a family makes a dutiful Christmas visit to their elderly grandmother, Peege, who is ending her life in a nursing home. They chatter superficially to cover the embarrassment of severely restricted communication. As they are leaving the eldest grandson stays behind and tries again, talking of their shared experiences in the past. Peege understands and is understood. With careful preparation and follow-up, this film could be used to trigger discussion both on old age and on communication. Age range 14 + .

**Distributed by:** Edward Patterson Associates Ltd.

**Title:** **A QUESTION OF AIDS**

**Production details:** Video. Colour. 25 mins.
ILEA, 1987

**Synopsis:** Uses a discussion format, where young people formulate and ask questions about HIV infection and AIDS, and a specialist answers them. Focuses on factual information, and provides a positive and optimistic view of life and sexual relationships. A useful video for older teenagers.

**Distributed by:** ILEA

**Title:** **SEX AND SENSIBILITY**

**Production details:** Video. Colour. 26 mins.
Straightforward Productions, 1987, for the National Abortion Campaign.

**Synopsis:** A low-key, low-budget video narrated by Pepsi and Shirlie which illustrates the options available to young people when faced with an unplanned pregnancy. Strong emphasis is placed on the role of contraception in avoiding unwanted pregnancy and on the seriousness of abortion as a considered alternative. The video is made up of a series of informal conversations with young single mothers and women who have had an abortion, interspersed with interviews with counsellors, doctors and social workers.

**Distributed by:** Concord Films Council Ltd.

# Videos and Films

**Title:** **SEX EDUCATION**

**Production details:** Video. Colour. 3 films; 20 mins. each.
BBC, 1984

**Synopsis:** Three programmes designed to help answer children's questions about the biology of sex and its role in human development. Age range 8-10.
Growing
  Growth and learning are continuous, but babyhood and puberty are particularly important times. Growth often occurs at different rates.
Someone New
  Starts with the developing human embryo, and follows a mother through pregnancy and birth.
Life Begins
  Illustrates the difference between boys and girls, and covers puberty and conception.

**Distributed by:** BBC Enterprises Film Hire Library or can be recorded off-air by holders of the relevant licence.

**Title:** **SOMEBODY'S DAUGHTER (YOU IN THE 70's)**

**Production details:** 16mm. Black and white. 5 films; 25 mins. each.
ILEA Schools Television, 1978

**Synopsis:** A story in five episodes which raises many issues for discussion around the themes of personal relationships, pregnancy and its consequences, mixed race marriages, and single parent families. Notes accompany. Age range 15 + .
Proof Positive
  Mandy Lewis is pregnant by Winston, who is black. Mrs Lewis wants Mandy to have an abortion, but Mandy wants to keep the baby.
Bangarang
  Winston's parents talk to him about the problems of marrying a white girl. How can he support a wife without a job or qualifications? Many has trouble trying to find somewhere to live.
It's a Mug's Game
  Mandy goes to maternity classes, thinks about adoption, and gets advice from Winston's mother. Winston mugs an elderly West Indian so he can buy Mandy a new pram.
One Home, One Away
  Mandy has her baby, and Winston is arrested. The court sends him to a detention centre. Later, a distraught Mandy abandons her daughter.
The Wife Wants a Child
  A girl finds the baby in a telephone kiosk, and takes it to the police station. Eventually a happy solution is found; Mandy gets someone to look after her baby, and Winston passes his exams in the detention centre.

**Distributed by:** Concord Films Council Ltd.
CFL Vision

**Title:** **STARTINGPOINT FILMS: THINKING ABOUT CONFLICT**

**Production details:** 16mm, video. Colour. 3 films; total running time 21 mins.
Broadside for Concord Films, 1983

**Synopsis:** Three short trigger films designed to promote discussion about conflict and conflict resolution, and indirectly about racism and sexism. Teaching pack accompanies. Age range 15 + .
The Party (8 mins.)
  As young people arrive at a party, tensions and jealousies soon become apparent. All goes well until a neighbour storms in and asks the teenagers to quieten down.

# Videos and Films

The Fight (4 mins.)
A playground fight erupts between two girls. Why did it happen? How should it have been resolved?

The Job (9 mins.)
Sophie is thinking about joining the police cadets, but meets opposition from the careers teacher, from her father, who thinks it an unsuitable training for girls, and from her friends.

**Distributed by:** Concord Films Council Ltd.

**Title:** **SWEET SIXTEEN AND PREGNANT**
**Production details:** 16mm, video. Colour. 29 mins. American.
Film Inc. USA, 1982
**Synopsis:** Several case studies present the options open to pregnant teenage girls — marriage, single parenthood, adoption, abortion. The emotions of the girls involved are vividly portrayed, and the film ends by suggesting that girls need not be pressured into sexual activity. Age range 15 + .
**Distributed by:** Educational Media International

**Title:** **TAKING CHANCES**
**Production details:** 16mm, Video. Colour. 22 mins. Canadian.
Mobius International for Ortho Pharmaceuticals, 1979
**Synopsis:** In a number of lively, dramatised sequences interspersed with discussion, young people explore why many sexually active teenagers do not use contraception. The film concentrates on attitudes rather than on giving information, although in a rather rambling interview with a birth control counsellor, the pill and condom plus foam are demonstrated. The need for responsibility and good communication are stressed throughout the film. Age range 15 + .
**Distributed by:** Concord Films Council Ltd.

**Title:** **TEENAGE FATHER**
**Production details:** 16mm. Colour. 30 mins. American.
National Children's Society of California, 1979
**Synopsis:** John is 17 years old and about to become a father. He is confident that offering the baby for adoption is the right thing to do, but his 15 year old girlfriend is not so sure. Through documentary-style interviews of the couple alone and together, with their respective parents, a counsellor, and some of John's friends we see John and Kim slowly coming to terms with the implications of parenthood. An excellent film for stimulating discussion on many aspects of relationships with friends and family and on pregnancy and parenting. Age range 15 + .
**Distributed by:** Concord Films Council Ltd.

**Title:** **THEN ONE YEAR (British Version)**
**Production details:** 16mm, video. Colour. 21 mins
Churchill Films, USA. British version produced by Boulton-Hawker Films 1978
**Synopsis:** Looks at the physiological changes in boys and girls at the onset of puberty, and the emotional worries which sometimes accompany these changes. Individual differences in growth rate, menstrual cycle etc. are shown to be normal. Good for use with mixed groups. Age range 11 + .
**Distributed by:** Boulton-Hawker Films Ltd.
Concord Films Council Ltd.
National Audio-Visual Aids Library

# Videos and Films

**Title:** **TRUE ROMANCE ETC.**

**Production details:** 16mm, video. Colour. 35 mins.
Newsreel Collective, 1981

**Synopsis:** An improvised film made with a multi-racial group of young people, which sets out to challenge sexist attitudes and stereotypes. More about the 'etc' than about romance, the film is built round events leading up to, and at, a party, and interwoven with interviews in which young people talk about their experience of gender stereotyping, being gay and about their relationships with friends and with the opposite sex. Could be useful for opening up discussion on many aspects of relationships and sexuality. Age range 15 + .

**Distributed by:** Concord Films Council Ltd.
The Other Cinema

**Title:** **US GIRLS**

**Production details:** Video. Black and white. 30 mins.
Albany Video Project, 1979

**Synopsis:** 'Us Girls' is a video adaptation of a play by the Albany Youth Theatre. It presents situations in the lives of five white girls from South London as they come up against sexist attitudes from parents, employers, boyfriends and each other. Not multi-cultural, but could be used by some groups of young teenagers, particularly girls' groups, as a discussion starter. Age range 15 + .

**Distributed by:** Albany Video

**Title:** **WHY IS IT FOR THEM . . . AND NOT ME?**

**Production details:** Video. Colour. Maureen's Story 24 mins., Jim's Story 25 mins., John's Story 15 mins., Elaine's Story 21 mins.
BAC Education and Publications Unit, 1984

**Synopsis:** In this video, four physically handicapped young adults speak bravely and frankly about the effect their various disabilities have had on their personal and sexual development. They come from a variety of backgrounds, range in age from 20 to 35, and have reached very different stages of personal fulfilment, but all speak movingly about their needs and hopes. The video is intended to raise the subject of sexuality and the physically handicapped for discussion by counsellors, teachers, doctors, nurses, occupational therapists, social workers etc., but could also be used to trigger discussion amongst disabled groups and their families. Extensive notes accompany.

**Distributed by:** Brook Advisory Centres Education and Publications Unit

# Additional resources (in alphabetical order)

**Title:** **ABORTION**

**Description:** A5 booklet. Revised 1983.

Contains questions and answers, statistics, and suggestions for further thought or study. Age range 16 + .

**Available from:** Brook Advisory Centres Education and Publications Unit

**Title:** **AIDS EDUCATION FOR SCHOOLS**

**Description:** 56-page teachers' Handbook, two card games, 10 laminated A4 pupil worksheets, 5 laminated A4 OHP masters, 1 laminated A3 factsheet.
Eastern Health and Social Services Board and Northern Ireland Council for Education Development (NICED), 1987

A helpful teaching package from Northern Ireland made up of three units containing two lessons each. Unit 1 situates AIDS firmly within the context of infectious diseases and could be used in biology or integrated science classes. Unit 2 clarifies information about AIDS and Unit 3 explores attitudes and values. Educators would need to provide a local checklist of useful addresses and reference to 'HIV' rather than 'the AIDS virus' would have to be preferable but the approach is participatory and open-ended and the package could be used by educators from a number of different disciplines.

**Available from:** Longman Resources Unit

**Title:** **AIDS. YOUNG ADULTS PROJECT PACK**

**Description:** Pack containing teachers' notes, six project cards, a wallchart, true or false factsheet, risk quiz, action plan, quiz on self-protection and a general list of information with space for local services to be added.
Lynda Jones, 1987

A useful pack for work with older teenagers, which encourages them to clarify information and explore attitudes but which also personalises the issue of HIV/AIDS by asking them to look closely at their own sexual behaviour. Emphasises that responsibility for transmission of the virus lies with individuals and that it is, therefore, possible to exercise control over one's sexual health.

**Available from:** AIDS Project Pack, East Berkshire Health Authority Health Promotion Unit.

**Title:** **ALL RIGHT FOR SOME**

**Description:** 96-page A4 workbook by Jane L. Thompson.
Century Hutchinson Ltd., 1986.

A workbook which uses cartoons, pictures and people's actual words to help young people look at their own prejudices and attitudes towards inequality between the sexes. As well as discussing stereotyped images of women, the book takes a hard look at equal pay and equal rights and makes a brief survey of the women's movement. There is a helpful 'useful addresses' section at the back of the book.

**Available from:** Booksellers

**Title:** **CHANGING IMAGES**

**Description:** 32-page, A4 collection of drawings in booklet form by Natalie Ninvalle, 1984

A collection of anti-sexist and anti-racist drawings which can be photocopied for use in schools and youth and community centres. The quality of some of the drawings is debatable, but they portray a positive and much needed alternative to the stereotyped images which confront most young people in their daily lives.

**Available from:** Sheba Feminist Publishers

# Additional resources

Additional resources

**Title:** **CHILDHOOD**

**Description:** 168-page, A4, Loose-leaf pack in a ring binder.
Dorit Braun and Naomi Eisenstadt, 1985

A pack designed to support teachers, trainers and other professionals working with adolescents or young families, which involves experiential and participatory learning around three major themes — 'Identity', 'Practical Experiences with Young Children', and 'Child, School and the Community'. The pack also contains an introductory section on getting a course underway, ideas on evaluation, a selection of reading and a resource list. Many of the activities and methods used in this excellent and innovative training resource can be adapted for use with young people.

**Available from:** The Open University

**Title:** **DISCUSSION CARDS**

**Description:** Ten laminated 'situation' cards, each with a separate sheet of questions for discussion, teachers' notes, resource list. 1986.

The situations described on the cards raise such issues as independence and trust, unwanted sex, parental roles, unplanned pregnancy, teenage marriage, sexually transmitted infections, sexual abuse and sexual harassment. The questions set which accompany encourage further exploration of each issue. Suitable for small group work.
Age range 14 + .

**Available from:** Brook Advisory Centre Education and Publications Unit

**Title:** **DIVORCE AND CHILDREN**

**Description:** 3 leaflets and a briefing paper in a plastic wallet. All items can also be purchased separately. 1988.

A simple but helpful pack for anyone working directly or indirectly with families experiencing separation and divorce. Of the three leaflets in the pack. 'Divorce and You' is for young people and is designed to help them sort out some of their feelings about divorce and explain some of the legal terms they may hear. The others two leaflets are for parents and counsellors respectively, while the briefing paper sets out the historical and sociological background to divorce and the research into its effects, particularly on children. Useful for any educator with pastoral responsibilities.

**Available from:** The Children's Society

**Title:** **DOING THINGS IN AND ABOUT THE HOME**

**Description:** Set of 24 black and white, A5 photographs, plus teachers' booklet. 1983.

Designed to stimulate discussion about sex roles, these photographs can also be used to focus attention on many other issues such as work and leisure, childhood, growing up, and equality. The teachers' booklet is full of ideas about how to use the photographs with children throughout the primary and secondary age-range.

**Available from:** Maidenhead Teachers' Centre

# Additional resources

**Title:** **FAMILY LIFESTYLES**
**Description:** 167-page, A4, loose-leaf pack in a ring-binder.
Dorit Braun and Naomi Eisenstadt, 1985.

A pack designed to support teachers, trainers and other professionals working with adolescents or young families. The materials encourage active learning around three major themes connected with family life education — 'What is a Family?', 'Social Roles' and 'Family Relationships'. There is also an introductory section on getting a course underway, ideas on evaluation, a selection of readings and a resources list. Although designed as a training pack, many of the activities and methods used can be adapted for use with young people. The photopack which comes with the pack is available for purchase separately (see 'What is a Family?').

**Distributed by:** The Open University

**Title:** **FIT FOR LIFE**
**Description:** Level 2 (9-13 years) 94 worksheets, teachers' notes.
Level 3 (13 + ) 116 worksheets, teachers' notes.
Schools Council/Health Education Authority, 1983.

Designed for slow learners aged 5-16, these materials are an extension of the Schools Council/HEC Health Education Project 5-13. Relationships are seen within the broad context of health education. The overall aims of the project are to foster positive self-esteem, to encourage the development of decision-making skills, and to help young people cope with the physical and mental changes which occur as they grow.

**Available from:** Macmillan Education

**Title:** **FPA CONTRACEPTIVE DISPLAY KIT**
**Description:** A kit containing a packet of contraceptive pills, an intra-uterine device (IUD), a diaphragm or cap, a tube of spermicide, a packet of vaginal pessaries, two condoms, an aerosol container of contraceptive foam and an applicator, a contraceptive sponge. Contents of kit revised 1985.

Useful for display and for small group discussion. Suitable for use with activity number 77: *Using the contraceptive kit.*

**Available from:** FPA Education Unit

**Title:** **FPIS LEAFLETS**
**Description:** The Family Planning Information Service (FPIS) provides a comprehensive range of leaflets on all aspects of family planning and related subjects (including sexually transmitted diseases). Posters and fact sheets are also available free of charge. Order form available. For the educator.

**Available from:** Family Planning Information Service

**Title:** **GENDER EQUALITY**
**Description:** 52-page, A4 spiral-bound book containing teachers' guidelines with photocopy masters of worksheets and pictures. 1986.

A flexible pack of twelve units designed to help primary school children confront and challenge gender bias in various aspects of everyday life. The activities are clearly and simply laid out and encourage pupils to examine language, jobs, books, comics, advertisements and the school environment. Preliminary and follow-up material adds to the versatility of the resource.

**Available from:** LDA.

# Additional resources

Title:            **GENDERWATCH!**

Description:       268-page, looseleaf A4 ring-binder. Devised by Kate Myers for the Equal Opportunities Commission and School Curriculum Development Committee, 1987.

A pack in three stages to help teachers, heads of department and head teachers to assess the current situation, devise strategies and monitor outcomes with regard to gender equality in their schools. A very flexible, non-judgemental resource which consists largely of self-assessment schedules to be filled in. Stage 1 invites the setting of goals and priorities, Stage 2 encourages observation of such issues as assemblies, movement around the school and text books and Stage 3 looks in detail at 21 different subject areas. A positive and objective way forward for any school concerned about gender.

Available from:   SCDC Publications

Title:            **THE GRAPEVINE GAME**

Description:       Boardgame for 2-8 players. 1984.

Used sensitively in small groups where there is an atmosphere of positive support and trust, this game could be a helpful and stimulating resource. Perhaps best suited to the later stages of a course when participants are comfortable sharing information and voicing opinions about all aspects of sexuality. Adequate preparation by the group leader is essential in case (s)he does not wish to use all the cards. Age range 16 + .

Available from:   New Grapevine

Title:            **GREATER EXPECTATIONS**

Description:       196-page book by Tricia Szirom and Sue Dyson. British edition edited by Hazel Slavin, 1986.

A substantial book of activities designed to raise awareness and self-esteem amongst girls and young women. Contains a theoretical framework, opportunities for values clarification, skills and confidence building exercises and lists for further resources.

Available from:   LDA.

Title:            **GROWING UP**

Description:       Four colour charts (38 × 51cm) plus teachers' notes, 1987.

Three of the charts in this set illustrate body changes at puberty for both boys and girls and periods. The fourth introduces a range of different 'characters' which are fleshed out in the teachers' notes with the aim of stimulating discussion on the emotional side of puberty.

Available from:   Pictorial Charts Education Trust

Title:            **HEALTH ACTION PACK**

Description:       Pack containing 192-page 'Health Activities Pack', 56-page book of Background Papers, Photopack of 32 black and white photos, A2 folding games board and A5 game cards. Gay Gray and Faith Hill for the Health Education Authority, 1988.

A flexible resource pack designed to help 16-19 year olds identify their own and the group's health needs and to increase their awareness of wider social and environmental issues. The Health Activities Book has eleven sections, each concerned with a different active learning method (i.e. working with groups, brainstorming, using printed materials, case studies, photographs, quizzes etc.).

# Additional resources

Each method is explained and specific examples, including some for use in work on relationships and sexuality, are given for each method. The Background Papers are a source of information for anyone working with 16-19 year olds on such topics as sexuality education and HIV and AIDS. Other support materials include a Photopack and Games Pack. All the materials have been extensively tried and tested in the field and provide an excellent springboard for further work in personal, social and health education in a wide variety of settings.

**Available from:** National Extension College

**Title:** **HEALTH EDUCATION 3-18**
**Description:** A comprehensive teaching pack containing pupil material and teachers' notes. 19 units divided into three levels according to age range (13-18). Schools Council/Health Education Authority, 1982.
*Please note:* individual units cannot be purchased separately.
The following units cover aspects of relationships and sexuality:
Level 1 (13-14 years)
   Coming of age (coping with change, puberty)
Level 2 (14-16 years)
   What would you do . . . about sexually transmitted diseases?
   You in a group (working in a group)
Level 3 (16 + )
   Health and self (self-profiling, mixing with new people)

**Available from:** Holmes McDougall Ltd.

**Title:** **HEALTH MATTERS**
**Description:** Pack consisting of 5 spiral-bound A4 booklets, a handbook for trainers, two posters. Christine Beels for the Health Education Authority, 1986.

A pack originally developed for use with YTS trainees but flexible enough to be used in other settings with 16-19 year olds. 'Stepping Out' is the title of the module on relationships. It contains 18 exercises exploring a wide variety of issues from stereotyping, body image, sexual identity and vocabulary, upbringing and families through to contraception, STDs, sexual pressure, expectations and love. Lively, thought-provoking material which has been extensively tried and tested in the field.

**Available from:** National Extension College

**Title:** **HEC PREGNANCY BOOK**
**Description:** A 79-page, A4 booklet. Free. Health Education Authority, 1984.

This booklet was designed to be given free of charge to first time mothers in the UK. Full of helpful information about pregnancy and the days immediately following the birth. For the educator.

**Available from:** Your local Health Education Unit, or single copies by post from Pregnancy Book, P.O. Box 416, London SE99 6YE. Further copies can be purchased from National Extension College.

**Title:** **IT HAPPENS TO US ALL**
**Description:** Teaching pack containing slide set, teachers' notes, pupil booklets, worksheets and samples, 1983.

A helpful teaching pack which looks at most of the physiological changes taking place during puberty. Designed to be used with mixed groups. Johnson and Johnson products feature heavily whenever menstruation is mentioned. Age range 10 + .

**Available from:** Johnson and Johnson

# Additional resources

**Title:** **IT'S YOUR LIFE: BABIES AND PARENTS**

**Description:** A4 booklet containing the comic strip 'It'll Never be the Same', plus additional pupil material. 1983.

The comic strip illustrates the problems encountered by a young couple trying to adapt to life with a new baby. Follow-up material includes an information file, and ideas for discussion and creative work. Age range 14 + .

**Available from:** Longman Resources Unit


**Title:** **IT'S YOUR LIFE: SEX AND BIRTH CONTROL**

**Description:** A4 booklet, containing the comic strip 'Don't Rush Me', plus additional pupil material. 1983.

The comic strip illustrates the dilemma of a girl whose boyfriend is putting pressure on her to have sex with him. She neither feels 'ready', nor has any knowledge of contraception. Follow-up material includes information and statistics about teenage pregnancies, one-parent families, the menstrual cycle and birth control, as well as questions for discussion and ideas for further work. Age range 15 + .

**Available from:** Longman Resources Unit


**Title:** **IT'S YOUR LIFE: SEX ROLES**

**Description:** A4 booklet, containing the comic strip 'It's Only Fair', plus additional pupil material. 1983.

The comic strip illustrates the changing roles of men and women at work and in their relationships. Follow-up material includes an information file, and ideas for discussion and creative work. Age range 14 + .

**Available from:** Longman Resource Unit


**Title:** **LIFE BEFORE BIRTH**

**Description:** Large colour chart (76 × 100cm) with notes. 1984.

In this chart, a combination of colour photographs and drawings are used to illustrate the development of the foetus within the uterus (intercourse and fertilisation are not shown). Notes accompany. For secondary pupils.

**Available from:** Pictorial Charts Educational Trust


**Title:** **LIFESKILLS TEACHER PROGRAMMES No. 1, No. 2, No. 3, No. 4**

**Description:** Four loose-leaf manuals of activities for young people, and notes for educators. 1979, 1982, 1986, 1988.

These materials are based on the belief that an information-centred approach does not encourage personal development as effectively as experiential and participatory learning. The emphasis is on developing a young person's ability to say 'I can. . . .' as well as 'I know. . . .' Lifeskills covered included 'How to be positive about oneself'. 'How to communicate effectively', and 'How to make, keep and end a relationship' (Programme No. 1); 'How to give and receive feedback' and 'How to learn from experience' (Programme No. 2); 'How to make decisions' and 'How to be an effective parent of young children' (Programme No. 3); 'Sexism cramps your style' and 'How to manage conflict (Programme No. 4). Age range 14 + .

**Available from:** Lifeskills Associates

# Additional resources

**Title:** **LIFE (TALKING POINTS, SET 2)**

**Description:** Set of 25 black and white photocards (20 × 30cm) with discussion points on the reverse of each card and teachers' guidelines. 1980.

Designed to aid language development in health and sex education in the primary school, these cards illustrate love and affection in human relationships, physical differences between males and females, intercourse, pregnancy, birth and the care of babies. All of the photographs except one feature white families.

**Available from:** Winslow Press Ltd.

**Title:** **LIVING CHOICES**

**Description:** Teachers' notes, 32-page workbook, spirit masters. 1976.

This resource takes young people through the variety of patterns of home life that are possible, and encourages them to explore their own attitudes and needs, and the implications of the choices they make. Age range 14 + .

**Available from:** CRAC Publications

**Title:** **MALE AND FEMALE**

**Description:** 15 laminated A4 cards. 1983.

These cards show illustrations of both the male and female sexual organs, the process of fertilisation and of pregnancy (they do not cover intercourse nor contraception). The illustrations are clearly headed and labelled, and can be used or displayed in any order. Probably best suited to small group work because of their A4 size.

**Available from:** FPA Education Unit

**Title:** **MALE AND FEMALE**

**Description:** Teachers' notes, 40-page workbook, spirit masters. Revised 1982.

This resource looks at the changing roles of men and women, and encourages young people to explore their own attitudes towards gender stereotyping. Age range 14 + .

**Available from:** CRAC Publications

**Title:** **ROLES, RELATIONSHIPS, RESPONSIBILITIES**

**Description:** A pack of 48 black and white, A4, trigger drawings. Chris Abuk for the Lambeth Health Education Project, 1982.

Drawings of a wide range of open-ended and multi-ethnic situations designed to trigger discussion. No written information or questions are attached to the drawings in order to encourage a variety of interpretations. Suitable for group work. Age range 13 + .

**Available from:** ILEA Learning Resource Branch

**Title:** **SAMPLE EDUCATION PACK**

**Description:** 16-page, A4 booklet for teachers, 3 pocket-sized booklets, A4 drawing of female pelvic and reproductive organs, details of school lecture service. Tampax Education Service, 1985.

The booklet for teachers, 'A Teaching Guide to Menstrual Health', provides helpful background information on menstruation. The pocket-sized booklets vary; one includes the facts about puberty and menstruation in a chatty, easy to read story, another provides a straightforward account of the major physiological changes at puberty, and the third is for mothers. Class sets of these booklets are available on request. If used by educators who are sensitive to different cultural needs, and who are aware that Tampax are not the only producers of sanitary protection in the British market, the pack could prove a useful supplement to other resources on puberty and menstruation.

**Available from:** Tampax Education Service. Free.

207

# Additional resources

**Title:** **SEXUALITY AND THE MENTALLY HANDICAPPED**

**Description:** Nine sets of slides, each with accompanying script. Winifred Kempton, 1978.

These slides are designed to be used with mentally handicapped young people. They are extremely comprehensive, and could provide the basis of a broad programme of sex education and personal relationships running over many months or years. The titles of the nine parts are:

Part 1 — Parts of the body
Part 2 — Male puberty
Part 3 — Female puberty
Part 4 — Social Behaviour
Part 5 — Human Reproduction
Part 6 — Birth Control
Part 7 — Venereal disease and sexual health
Part 8 — Marriage
Part 9 — Parenting

**Available from:** Can be hired from FPA Education Unit, SPOD and local health education/ promotion units.


**Title:** **TEACHING ABOUT HIV AND AIDS**

**Description:** 44-page, A4 ring-binder containing 16 lesson outlines, 10 photocopiable worksheets, 3 trigger cartoon strips, leaflets and factsheets for teachers, useful addresses and a reading list. Health Education Authority, 1988.

A pack divided into three modules for use with 12-13 year olds, 14-15 year olds and 16 + . Each module is designed to help young people clarify information about HIV and AIDS and explore attitudes and values. Guidelines for a parents/ governors evening workshop are also included.

**Available from:** Local Health Education/Promotion Units
In case of difficulty, contact the Health Education Authority.


**Title:** **TEACHING ABOUT STD**

**Description:** Four A4, spiral-bound booklets in a plastic folder. 1985.

The four booklets are entitled 'Introduction and Objectives', 'Facts and Figures' and 'Pupil Material and Worksheets'. The emphasis is on correcting misinformation about STDs, and the educator is given clear and helpful notes to back up the pupil material. Exercises include knowledge quizzes and a role-play in which a specialist planning team on STDs meet to discuss what, if any, local action should be taken. Age range 15 + .

**Available from:** Department of Health Education and Promotion,
Doncaster Health Authority.


**Title:** **THINK WELL (9-13)**

**Description:** A comprehensive teaching pack made up of a teachers' guide, 24 copyright-free spirit masters, and resource sheets. All three items can be purchased separately. Schools Council/Health Education Council, 1977.

The 'Think Well' materials are part of the Schools Council/HEC Health Education Project (5-13). The most relevant units for work on relationships and sexuality are Unit 1: Myself (self concept, growth and sexual development) and Unit 2: One of Many (relationships, puberty, intercourse and reproduction). The eight units in the Teachers' Guide can only be purchased as a set. Age range 9-13.

**Available from:** Thomas Nelson and Sons Ltd.

# Additional resources

**Title:** **TIME OF THE MONTH**

**Description:** A boardgame for 2-12 players plus comprehensive User's Notes, 1987.

A game designed to help young women glean further information and share opinions and feelings about menstruation. Players throw a dice to move round the board and pick up 'True/False' or 'Action' cards along the way which contain questions to answer or points for discussion. A positive way of encouraging young women to share what they know and admit their fears about periods, fertility and contraception. Age range 14 + .

**Available from:** National Association of Youth Clubs

**Title:** **UNDERSTANDING OTHERS**

**Description:** 20 laminated, A4 cards, with trigger questions on the reverse side, plus teachers' notes. 1980.

Case studies on aspects of adolescence and personal relationships. Each card requires a reasonable level of literacy. Age range 14 + .

**Available from:** TACADE

**Title:** **WHAT IS A FAMILY?**

**Description** Set of 22 black and white, A5 photographs, plus 24-page booklet for the educator. Naomi Eisenstadt and Dorit Braun, 1985.

The booklet provides helpful ideas for activities based around the photographs, while the photographs themselves are lively, varied and culturally diverse. Suitable for group work on the affective and emotional aspects of family life. Can be used with young people and adults.

**Available from:** Development Education Centre

**Title:** **WHO ARE YOU STARING AT?**

**Description:** 36 black and white photoposters, 6 booklets, audio-cassette, teachers' notes. Community Service Volunteers and Mental Health Film Council, 1980.

In this photopack, six young disabled people talk about their lives, the problems they face, and their relationships with family and friends. A flexible resource which aims to help dispel prejudices about people who are different, and to encourage an open, sensitive outlook towards disability.

**Available from:** Community Service Volunteers.

**Title:** **WHY DISCUSS ABORTION?**

**Description:** Teaching pack containing a factsheet exercise, three factchecks, 4 case studies, a role-play and a resource list. 1984.

A helpful pack providing information and discussion material about abortion. Sensitive both to the controversy surrounding abortion and to the dilemmas facing young people. Age range 16 + .

**Available from:** Abortion Law Reform Association (ALRA)

**Title:** **WORKING WITH UNCERTAINTY**

**Description:** 50-page, A4 training manual. Hilary Dixon and Peter Gordon for the FPA Education Unit and AIDS Education Unit, Cambridge Health Authority, 1987.

A manual for all educators who have received some HIV/AIDS awareness training themselves and wish to go back to their work setting and train others. It offers exercises and materials to help participants consider their feelings and attitudes, share their difficulties and practise communication skills. Could boost knowledge levels and confidence amongst educators if introduced by a colleague with experience of HIV/Aids training.

**Available from:** FPA Education Unit

# Useful addresses

**ABORTION LAW REFORM ASSOCIATION (ALRA)**
88 Islington High Street
London N1 8EG
Tel: 01-359 5200

**ALBANY TRUST**
24 Chester Square
London SW1W 9HS
Tel: 01-730 5871
(Advice and counselling on personal relationships)

**ALBANY VIDEO**
Distribution
Douglas Way
London SE8 4AG
Tel: 01-692 6322

**BBC ENTERPRISES FILM HIRE LIBRARY**
6 Royce Road
Peterborough PE1 5YB
Tel: 0733-315315

**BEAUMONT SOCIETY**
BM Box 3084
London WC1V 6XX
(Advice and counselling on gender identity)

**BOULTON-HAWKER FILMS LTD.**
Hadleigh
Ipswich
Suffolk IP7 5BG
Tel: 0473-822235

**BOUNTY VISION**
Bounty Services Ltd.
Diss
Norfolk IP22 3HH
Tel: 0379-51081

**BRITISH ASSOCIATION FOR COUNSELLING (BAC)**
37A Sheep Street
Rugby
Warwickshire CV21 3BX
Tel: 0788-783328

**BRITISH PREGNANCY ADVISORY SERVICES (BPAS)**
Austy Manor
Wootton Wawen
Solihull
West Midlands
Tel: 05642-3225

**BROOK ADVISORY CENTRES**
153A East Street
London SE17 2SD
Tel: 01-708 1234

**BROOK ADVISORY CENTRES**
Education and Publication Unit
24 Albert Street
Birmingham B4 7UD
Tel: 021-643 1554

**CAMPAIGN FOR HOMOSEXUAL EQUALITY (CHE)**
274 Upper Street
London N1 2UA
Tel: 01-359 3973

**CATHOLIC MARRIAGE ADVISORY COUNCIL**
15 Lansdowne Road
London W11
Tel: 01-727 0141

**CENTRAL INDEPENDENT TELEVISION PLC**
Video Resources Unit
Central House
Broad Street
Birmingham B1 2JP
Tel: 021-643 9898

**CFL VISION**
P.O. Box 35
Wetherby
Yorks. SL23 7EX
Tel: 0937-541010

**CHILDREN'S SOCIETY**
The Publications Editor
Edward Rudolf House
Margery Street
London WC1X 0JL
Tel: 01-837 4299

**CINEMA OF WOMEN**
27 Clerkenwell Close
London EC1R 0AT
Tel: 01-251 4978

**CITIZENS' ADVICE BUREAUX**
Myddleton House
115-123 Pentonville Road
London N1 9LZ
Tel: 01-833 2181

**COMMUNITY SERVICE VOLUNTEERS**
237 Pentonville Road
London N1 9NJ
Tel: 01-278 6601

# Useful addresses

**CONCORD FILMS COUNCIL LTD.**
201 Felixstowe Road
Ipswich
Suffolk IP3 9BJ
Tel: 0473-726012/715754

**CONNEXIONS**
4th Floor
10-20 Dean Street
Newcastle Upon Tyne NE1 1PG
Tel: 0632-616581

**CRAC PUBLICATIONS**
Hobsons Press (Cambridge) Ltd.
Bateman Street
Cambridge CB2 1LZ
Tel: 0223-354551

**DEPT. OF HEALTH EDUCATION AND PROMOTION**
Doncaster Health Authority
Alverley Lodge
St. Catherine's Hospital
Tickhill Road
Doncaster
S. Yorks DN4 8QN
Tel: 0302-854661

**DEVELOPMENT EDUCATION CENTRE**
Selly Oak Colleges
Bristol Road
Birmingham B29 6LE
Tel: 021-472 3255

**DUREX CONTRACEPTION INFORMATION SERVICE**
North Circular Road
London E4 8QA
Tel: 01-527 2377

**EAST BERKSHIRE HEALTH AUTHORITY**
Health Promotion Unit
Frances House
Frances Road
Windsor
Berks. SL4 3DP
Tel: 07538-59221

**EDUCATIONAL MEDIA INTERNATIONAL**
25 Boileau Road
London W5 3AL
Tel: 01-998 8657

**EDWARD PATTERSON ASSOCIATES LTD.**
'Treetops'
Cannongate Road
Hythe
Kent CT21 5PT
Tel: 0303-64195

**EQUAL OPPORTUNITIES COMMISION (EOC)**
Quay Street
Manchester M3 3HN
Tel: 061-833 9244

**FAMILY PLANNING ASSOCIATION (FPA)**
27-35 Mortimer Street
London W1N 7RJ
Tel: 01-636 7866

**FAMILY PLANNING INFORMATION SERVICE (FPIS)**
27-35 Mortimer Street
London W1N 7RJ
Tel: 01-636 7866

**FPA EDUCATION UNIT**
27-35 Mortimer Street
London W1N 7RJ
Tel: 01-636 7866

**GAY SWITCHBOARD**
BM Switchboard
London WC1N 3XX
Tel: 01-837 7324

**GAY YOUTH MOVEMENT**
BM/GYM
London WC1N 3XX

**GLENBUCK FILMS LTD.**
Glenbuck Road
Surbiton
Surrey KT6 6BT
Tel: 01-399 0022

**GUILD SOUND & VISION**
6 Royce Road
Peterborough PE1 5YB
Tel: 0733-315315

**GRAVES MEDICAL AUDIOVISUAL LIBRARY**
Holly House
220 New London Road
Chelmsford
Essex CM2 9BJ
Tel: 0245-283351

**HEALTH EDUCATION AUTHORITY (HEA)**
(Formerly Health Education Council)
Hamilton House
Mabledon Place
London WC1H 9TX
Tel: 01-631 0930

## Useful addresses

**HOLMES McDOUGALL LTD.**
Allander House
137-141 Leith Walk
Edinburgh EH6 8NS
Tel: 031-554 9444

**ILEA LEARNING RESOURCES BRANCH**
Centre for Learning Resources
275 Kennington Lane
London SE11 5QZ
Tel: 01-633 5995 (for order queries)
01-622 9966 (for information)

**INCEST CRISIS LINE**
Tel: 01-890 4732/422 5100

**INTERNATIONAL PLANNED PARENTHOOD FEDERATION (IPPF)**
Regents College
Inner Circle
Regents Park
London NW1 4NS
Tel: 01-486 0741

**JOHNSON AND JOHNSON**
Schools Information Service
P.O. Box 3
Diss
Norfolk IP22 3HH

**LDA (LEARNING DEVELOPMENT AIDS)**
Duke Street
Wisbech
Cambs. PE13 2AE
Tel: 0945-63441

**LESBIAN LINE**
BM Box 1514
London WC1N 3XX
Tel: 01-251 6911

**LIFESKILLS ASSOCIATES**
Clarendon Chambers
51 Clarendon Road
Leeds LS2 9NZ
Tel: 0532-467128

**LONGMAN RESOURCES UNIT**
62 Hallfield Road
Layerthorpe
York
Yorkshire YO3 7XQ
Tel: 0904-425444

**MACMILLAN EDUCATION**
Houndmills
Basingstoke
Hampshire RG21 2XS
Tel: 0256-29242

**MAIDENHEAD TEACHERS' CENTRE**
St. Edmund's House
Ray Mill Road West
Maidenhead SL6 8SB
Tel: 0628-27467

**MARIE STOPES HOUSE**
The Well Woman Centre
108 Whitfield Street
London W1
Tel: 01-388 0662

**MIRROR VISION VIDEO**
Mirror Group Newspapers
Holborn Circus
London EC1
Tel: 01-353 0246

**NATIONAL AIDS HELPLINE**
Tel: 0800-567 123

**NATIONAL ASSOCIATION FOR YOUNG PERSONS'S COUNSELLING AND ADVISORY SERVICES (NAYPCAS)**
17-23 Albion Street
Leicester LE1 66D
Tel: 0533-554775 Ext. 22/36

**NATIONAL ASSOCIATION OF YOUTH CLUBS**
Keswick House
30 Peacock Lane
Leicester LE1 5NY
Tel: 0533-29514

**NATIONAL AUDIO-VISUAL AIDS LIBRARY**
The George Building
Normal College
Bangor
Gwynedd LL57 2PZ
Tel: 0248-370144

**NATIONAL CHILDBIRTH TRUST (NCT)**
9 Queensborough Terrace
London W2
Tel: 01-221 3833

**NATIONAL CHILDREN'S BUREAU**
8 Wakley Street
London EC1V 9QE
Tel: 01-278 9441

# Useful addresses

**NATIONAL COUNCIL FOR ONE PARENT FAMILIES**
255 Kentish Town Road
London NW5
Tel: 01-267 1361

**NATIONAL EXTENSION COLLEGE**
18 Brooklands Avenue
Cambridge CB2 2HN
Tel: 0223-316644

**NATIONAL MARRIAGE GUIDANCE COUNCIL (Now called RELATE)**
Herbert Gray College
Little Church Street
Rugby
Warwickshire
Tel: 0788-73241

**NATIONAL SOCIETY FOR THE PREVENTION OF CRUELTY TO CHILDREN (NSPCC)**
1 Riding House Street
London W1
Tel: 01-580 8812

**NATIONAL YOUTH BUREAU**
17-23 Albion Street
Leicester LE1 66D
Tel: 0533-554775

**NEW GRAPEVINE**
Sex Education Project
416 St John Street
London EC1V 4NJ
Tel: 01-278 9147

**THE OPEN UNIVERSITY**
Learning Materials Service
Centre of Continuing Education
P.O. Box 188
Milton Keynes
MK7 6DH
Tel: 0908-74066

**THE OTHER CINEMA**
79 Wardour Street
London W1V 3TH
Tel: 01-734 8508/9

**PARENTS ANONYMOUS**
6 Manor Gardens
London N7 6LA
Tel: 01-263 8918
(For parents in crisis situations)

**PICTORIAL CHARTS EDUCATION TRUST**
27 Kirchen Road
London W13 0UD
Tel: 01-567 5343/9206

**PREGNANCY ADVISORY SERVICES (PAS)**
11 Charlotte Street
London W1
Tel: 01-637 8962

**RAPE CRISIS CENTRE**
P.O. Box 69
London WC1X 9NJ
Tel: 01-278 3956 (office)/837 1600 (24 hour emergency)

**ROLF HARRIS VIDEO LTD.**
43 Drury Lane
London WC2B 5RT
Tel: 01-240 8777

**SAMARITANS (Office & Administration)**
17 Uxbridge Road
Slough
Bucks.
Tel: 0753-32713

**SCDC PUBLICATIONS**
Newcombe House
45 Notting Hill Gate
London W11 3JB

**SEXUAL AND PERSONAL RELATIONSHIPS OF THE DISABLED (SPOD)**
286 Camden Road
London N7 0BJ
Tel: 01-607 8851

**SHEBA FEMINIST PUBLISHERS**
488 Kingsland Road
London E8 4AE
Tel: 01-254 1590

**TACADE (Teachers' Avisory Council on Alcohol and Drug Education)**
3rd Floor
Furness House
Trafford Road
Salford M5 2XJ
Tel: 061-848 0351

## Useful addresses

**TAMPAX EDUCATION SERVICE**
Tambrands Ltd.
Dunsbury Way
Havant
Hants PO9 5DG
Tel: 0705-474141

**TERRENCE HIGGINS TRUST**
BM AIDS
London WC1N 3XX
Tel: 01-831 0330 (admin.)
01-242 1010 (Helpline 3pm-10pm daily)

**THOMAS NELSON AND SONS LTD.**
Nelson House
Mayfield Road
Walton on Thames
Surrey KT12 5PL
Tel: 0932-246133

**WINSLOW PRESS LTD.**
Telford Road
Bicester
Oxon. OX6 0TS
Tel: 0869-244733

# Activity index

# Activity index/Activity acknowledgements

## Activity acknowledgements

3 Evaluation voting; 7 Telemessages; 36 The family — values voting; 37 The family — values ranking, based on activities in 'Values Clarification, A Handbook of Practical Strategies for Teachers and Students' by Simon, S., Howe, L., Kirschenbaum, H. (Hart, New York, 1978)

40 The problem page, from an idea in the 'Loving and Caring' Notes for Film Users.

47 How to say no . . ., from an idea suggested by Sol Gordon.

45 Decisions, decisions, developed from an activity in 'Values in Sexuality: A New Approach to Sex Education', Morrison, E. and Underhill Price, M. (Hart, New York, 1974)

48 Re-write the story, Bob and Carol, Ted and Alice, and Mrs Davis, developed from 'Discovering the Needs and Interests of Young People' with original permission from the Joint Board of Christian Education, Melbourne, 1980

55 What's in the bag? — collage, based on an idea in 'Education for Sexuality', Burt, J. and Meeks, L. (W. B. Saunders Company, Philadelphia, 1975)

92 Getting it together, based on an idea by Jane Dunstan.